SPRINGHOUSE

Professional Care Guide

Immune
Disorders

SPRINGHOUSE

Professional Care Guide

Immune Disorders

Springhouse Corporation
Springhouse, Pennsylvania

Staff

Senior Publisher
Matthew Cahill

Clinical Manager
Cindy Tryniszewski, RN, MSN

Art Director
John Hubbard

Senior Editor
June Norris

Editors
Edith McMahon, Elizabeth Weinstein

Clinical Editor
Judith E. Meissner, RN, MSN

Designers
Stephanie Peters (senior associate art director), Lynn Foulk (book designer)

Copy Editors
Cynthia Breuninger (manager), Lynette High, Doris Weinstock

Typography
Diane Paluba (manager), Elizabeth Bergman, Joyce Rossi Biletz, Phyllis Marron, Valerie Rosenberger

Manufacturing
Deborah C. Meiris (manager), Patricia Dorshaw, T.A. Landis

Production Coordinator
Patricia McCloskey

Editorial Assistants
Beverly Lane, Mary Madden, Dianne Tolbert

Indexer
Robin Hipple

The cover illustration depicts the body's cellular response to invading organisms. Illustration by Kevin A. Somerville.

---

for users of the Transactional Reporting Service is 0874347807/95 $00.00 + $.75.
Printed in the United States of America.

℟ A member of the Reed Elsevier plc group

PCG3-020695

Library of Congress Cataloging-in-Publication Data
Immunologic disorders.
    p. cm. — (Professional care guides)
Includes bibliographical references and index.
    1. Immunologic diseases — Nursing.
    2. Nursing care plans. I. Springhouse Corporation.
    II. Series.
[DNLM: 1. Immunologic Diseases.
WD 300 1995]
RC582.I464 1995
610.73'6 — dc20
DNLM/DLC   94-34606
ISBN 0-87434-780-7   CIP

Contents

Contributors and Consultants

Marlene M. Ciranowicz, RN, MSN, CDE
Independent Nurse Consultant
Dresher, Pa.

JoAnn Coleman, RN, MS, CS, OCN
Clinical Nurse Specialist, Gastrointestinal Surgery
The Johns Hopkins Hospital
Baltimore

Ellie Z. Franges, RN, MSN, CCRN, CNRN
Neuroscience Coordinator
Sacred Heart Hospital
Allentown, Pa.

Susan Galea, RN, MSN, CCRN
Surgical Intensive Care Unit Nurse
Hospital of the University of Pennsylvania
Philadelphia

Judith E. Meissner, RN, MSN
Independent Nurse Consultant
Warminster, Pa.

John J. O'Shea, MD
Chief, Lymphocyte Cell Biology Section
Arthritis and Rheumatism Branch
National Institute of Arthritis and Musculoskeletal
and Skin Diseases
National Institutes of Health
Bethesda, Md.

Brenda Shelton, RN, MS, CCRN, OCN
Critical Care Clinical Nurse Specialist
The Johns Hopkins Hospital
Baltimore

Foreword

Not so many years ago, when I would mention that I did research in immunology, my comment was usually met with a blank stare — as if I had spoken in a foreign language. Most people had little or no knowledge of immunology and how it related to human disease. Today, this has changed dramatically. The reason is obvious: AIDS.

However, despite the scientific and public attention to this deadly syndrome, the knowledge of many people — including those in the health professions — remains woefully incomplete. Although many are familiar with the concept of immunodeficiency and its implications, few appreciate the spectrum of phenomena that result in immunodeficiency or grasp the distinction between immunodeficiency and autoimmunity.

Moreover, rapid advances in immunology are forcing health care professionals to keep up-to-date with an ever-expanding knowledge base. Consider this: Assisted by recombinant DNA technology, researchers have successfully cloned many genes that govern the immune response. We now understand the structure and function of the proteins encoded by these genes.

In addition, answers to fundamental questions that have eluded researchers continue to surface. For instance, we now know the specific T- and B-cell structures that recognize foreign antigens. And we know the nature of antigens that are recognized by these two different types of cells.

What's more, molecular cloning has led to the identification of cytokines responsible for communication between immune cells. Recently, the molecular basis of several immunodeficiencies was identified, and gene therapy was initiated to treat severe combined immunodeficiency brought on by adenosine deaminase deficiency.

Despite so many advances, great gaps in our knowledge remain. For example, a molecular understanding of tolerance and anergy eludes us, and our understanding of autoimmune disorders remains relatively unsophisticated.

Nevertheless, we must effectively bring into our practices what we already know. Certainly AIDS alone makes this a requirement. But consider also that another immune disorder, rheumatoid arthritis, affects more than 10% of Americans over age 65 and 1% to 2% of the overall adult population. Even larger numbers of Americans—about 40 million in all—suffer from asthma and other allergic disorders. In fact, nearly 10% of all doctor's visits are spurred by allergies.

Keeping abreast of scientific advances and the practical applications of immunology would be a daunting task without a reference such as *Immune Disorders.* A part of the Professional Care Guide series, this reference provides authoritative, easy-to-use, and up-to-date information for any health care professional. It begins by examining the causes, diagnosis, and treatment of immune disorders. Subsequent chapters address allergies, autoimmune disorders, and AIDS and other immunodeficiencies. The book's extensive appendices cover organ-specific autoimmune disorders, chief complaints in immune disorders, immune drugs and treatments, and the *ICD-9-CM* classification of immune disorders.

For convenience, each disorder in the book is organized consistently. Each one covers causes, signs and symptoms, diagnostic studies, treatments, and special considerations. At the end of each chapter, you'll find a helpful self-test section. This section allows the reader to quickly evaluate his understanding of the chapter's main concepts and clinical issues. Answers to these questions and the rationales appear at the back of the book.

With all of these features, health care professionals will find this volume highly relevant and thorough. It quickly brings you up-to-date on immune disorders.

John J. O'Shea, MD
Chief, Lymphocyte Cell Biology Section
Arthritis and Rheumatism Branch
National Institute of Arthritis and Musculoskeletal
and Skin Diseases
National Institutes of Health
Bethesda, Md.

CHAPTER 1

Introduction

The environment contains thousands of pathogenic micro-organisms—viruses, bacteria, fungi, and parasites. Ordinarily, we protect ourselves from infectious organisms and other harmful invaders through an elaborate network of safeguards—the host defense system. Understanding how this system functions provides the framework for studying various immune disorders.

Host defenses

The host defense system includes physical and chemical barriers to infection, the inflammatory response, and the immune response. Physical barriers, such as the skin and mucous membranes, prevent invasion by most organisms. Those organisms that do penetrate this first line of defense simultaneously trigger the inflammatory and immune responses. Both responses involve cells derived from a hematopoietic stem cell in the bone marrow. (See *Understanding the immune response*, page 2.)

The inflammatory response involves polymorphonuclear leukocytes, basophils, mast cells, platelets and, to some extent, monocytes and macrophages. The immune response primarily involves the interaction of lymphocytes (T and B cells), macrophages, and macrophage-like cells and their products. These cells may be circulating or localized in the tissues and organs of the immune system, including the thymus, lymph nodes, spleen, and tonsils.

The thymus participates in the maturation of T lymphocytes (cell-mediated immunity); here these cells are "educated" to differentiate self from nonself. In contrast, B lymphocytes (humoral immunity) mature in the bone marrow. The key humoral effector mechanism is the production of immunoglobulin by B cells and the subsequent activation of the complement cascade. The lymph nodes, spleen, liver, and intestinal lymphoid tissue help remove and destroy circulating antigens in the blood and lymphatic system.

Understanding the immune response

When foreign substances invade the body, two types of immune responses reinforce white blood cells' defense: humoral and cell-mediated immunity. Both types involve lymphocytes that undergo differential development to become B cells and T cells.

Humoral immunity
In humoral immunity, antigens stimulate B cells to differentiate into plasma cells and produce circulating antibodies that destroy bacteria and viruses before they can enter host cells.

Cell-mediated immunity
In cell-mediated immunity, helper T cells spur B cells to manufacture antibodies.

Effector T cells kill antigens directly. Both helper and effector T cells produce lymphokines (proteins that induce an inflammatory response and mediate the delayed hypersensitivity reaction). Suppressor T cells regulate both humoral and cell-mediated immune responses.

Macrophages present antigens to B cells and T cells. This stimulates B cells to mature into antibody-producing plasma cells and sensitizes T cells, making them capable of interacting directly with the foreign material.

Each time foreign substances invade the body, T cells and B cells preserve a "memory" of the encounter, which provides long-term immunity to many diseases.

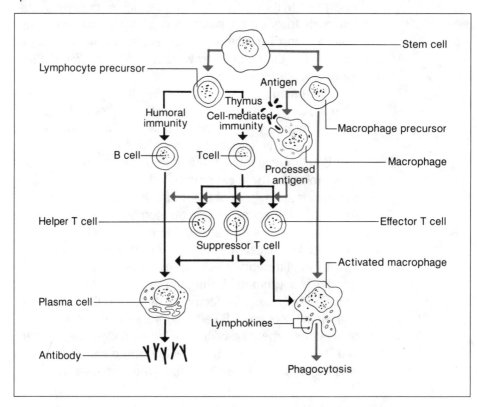

Major histocompatibility complex

The major histocompatibility complex (MHC) is a cluster of genes on human chromosome 6 that plays a pivotal role in the immune response. Also known as human leukocyte antigen (HLA) genes, these genes are inherited in an autosomal codominant manner. That is, each individual receives one set of MHC genes (haplotype) from each parent, and both sets of genes are expressed on the individual's cells. These genes play a role in the recognition of self versus nonself and the interaction of immunologically active cells by coding for cell-surface proteins.

Classifications

HLA antigens are divided into three classes. Class I antigens appear on nearly all of the body's cells and include the HLA-A, HLA-B, and HLA-C antigens. During tissue graft rejection, they are the chief antigens recognized by the host. When killer (CD8$^+$) T cells use a virally infected antigen, they recognize it in the context of a class I antigen.

Class II antigens only appear on B cells, macrophages, and activated T cells. They include the HLA-D and HLA-DR antigens. Class II antigens promote efficient collaboration between immunocompetent cells. CD4$^+$ (helper) T cells require that the antigen be presented in the context of a class II antigen. Because these antigens also determine whether an individual responds to a particular antigen, they're also known as immune response genes.

Class III antigens include certain complement (C) proteins (C2, C4, and factor B).

Antigens

Any substance that can induce an immune response is an antigen. T and B lymphocytes have specific receptors that respond to specific antigen molecular shapes (epitopes). In B cells, this receptor is an immunoglobulin (antibody) cell: immunoglobulin D (IgD) or IgM, sometimes referred to as a surface immunoglobulin. The T-cell antigen receptor recognizes antigens only in association with specific cell surface molecules known as the major histocompatibility complex (MHC). (See *Major histocompatibility complex.*) MHC molecules, which differ among individuals, identify substances as self or nonself. Slightly different antigen receptors can recognize a phenomenal number of distinct antigens, which are coded by distinct, variable region genes.

Groups, or clones, of lymphocytes exist with identical receptors for a specific antigen. The clone of lymphocytes rapidly proliferates when exposed to this specific antigen. Some of these lymphocytes further differentiate, and others become memory cells, which enable a more rapid response – the memory or anamnestic response – to a subsequent challenge by the antigen.

Many factors influence antigenicity. Among them are the physical or chemical characteristics of the antigen, its relative foreignness, and the individual's genetic makeup, particularly regarding the MHC molecules. Most antigens are large molecules, such as proteins or polysaccharides. (Smaller molecules, such as drugs, that aren't antigenic by themselves are known as haptens. These haptens can bind with larger molecules, or carriers, and become antigenic or immunogenic.) The relative foreignness of the antigen influences the intensity of the immune response. For example, little or no immune response may follow transfusion of serum proteins between humans; however, a vigorous immune response (serum sickness) often follows transfusion of horse serum proteins to a human. Genetic makeup may also determine why some individuals respond to certain antigens whereas others do not. The genes responsible for this phenomenon encode the MHC molecules.

B lymphocytes

Contributing factors in humoral immunity are B lymphocytes and their products, immunoglobulins. The binding of soluble antigen with B-cell antigen receptors initiates the humoral immune response. The activated B cells differentiate into plasma cells that secrete immunoglobulins, or antibodies. This response is regulated by T lymphocytes and their products, which are known as lymphokines. These lymphokines, which include interleukin-2 (IL-2), IL-4, IL-5, and interferon-8, are important in determining the class of immunoglobulin made by B cells.

The immunoglobulins secreted by plasma cells are four-chain molecules with two heavy and two light chains. (See *Structure of the immunoglobulin molecule.*) Each chain has a variable (V) region and one or more constant (C) regions coded for by separate genes. The V regions of both light and heavy chains participate in the binding of antigens. The C regions of the heavy chain provide a binding site for Fc receptors on cells and govern other mechanisms.

Any clone of B cells has one antigen specificity determined by the V regions of its light and heavy chains. However, the clone can change the class of immunoglobulin that it makes by changing the association between its V region genes and heavy chain, C region genes (a process known as isotype switching). For example, a clone of B cells geneti-

Structure of the immunoglobulin molecule

The immunoglobulin molecule consists of four polypeptide chains—two heavy (H) and two light (L) chains—held together by disulfide bonds. The H chain has one variable (V) and at least three constant (C) regions. The L chain has one V and one C region.

Together, the V regions of the H and L chains form a pocket known as the antigen-binding site. This site is located within the antigen-binding fragment (Fab) region of the molecule.

Part of the C region of the H chains forms the crystallizable fragment (Fc) region of the molecule. This region mediates effector mechanisms, such as complement activation, and is the portion of the immunoglobulin molecule bound by Fc receptors on phagocytic cells, mast cells, and basophils.

Each immunoglobulin molecule also has two antibody-combining sites (except for the immunoglobulin molecule, which has ten, and IgA, which may have two or more).

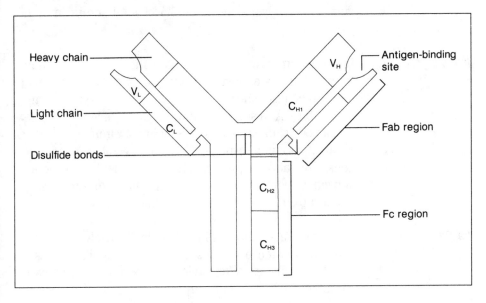

cally preprogrammed to recognize tetanus toxoid will first make an IgM antibody against tetanus toxoid and later an IgG or other antibody against it.

The known classes of immunoglobulins—IgG, IgM, IgA, IgE, and IgD—are distinguished by the constant portions of their heavy chains. However, each class has a kappa or a lambda light chain, which gives rise to many subtypes and provides the almost limitless combinations of light and heavy chains that give immunoglobulins their specificity.

Immunoglobulin G   The smallest immunoglobulin, IgG appears in all body fluids because of its ability to permeate membranes as a single structural unit (a monomer). It constitutes 75% of total serum immunoglobulins and is the major antibacterial and anti-viral antibody.

Immunoglobulin M   The largest immunoglobulin, IgM appears as a pentamer (five monomers joined by a J chain). Unlike IgG—which is produced mainly in the secondary, or recall, response—IgM dominates in the primary, or initial, immune response. But like IgG, IgM is involved in classic antibody reactions, including precipitation, agglutination, neutralization, and complement fixation. Because of its size, IgM cannot readily cross membrane barriers and is usually present only in the vascular system. IgM constitutes 5% of total serum immunoglobulins.

Immunoglobulin A   IgA exists in serum primarily as a monomer. In secretory form, IgA exists almost exclusively as a dimer (two monomer molecules joined by a J chain and a secretory component chain). As a secretory immunoglobulin, IgA defends external body surfaces and is present in colostrum, saliva, tears, nasal fluids, and respiratory, GI, and genitourinary secretions. This antibody is considered important in preventing antigenic agents from attaching to epithelial surfaces. IgA makes up 20% of total serum immunoglobulins.

Immunoglobulin E   Present in trace amounts in serum, IgE is involved in the release of vasoactive amines stored in basophils and tissue mast cell granules. When released, these bioamines cause the allergic effects characteristic of this type of hypersensitivity (erythema, itching, smooth-muscle contraction, secretions, and swelling).

Immunoglobulin D   Present as a monomer in serum in minute amounts, IgD is the predominant antibody found on the surface of B lymphocytes and serves mainly as an antigen receptor. It may function in controlling lymphocyte activation or suppression.

T lymphocytes   The chief participants in cell-mediated immunity are T lymphocytes and macrophages. Immature T lymphocytes are derived from the bone marrow but then migrate to the thymus; there they undergo a maturation process that is dependent on products of the MHC, human leukocyte antigen (HLA) genes. Thus, mature T cells can distinguish between self and nonself. T cells acquire certain surface molecules, or markers; these markers, combined with the T-cell antigen receptor, promote the particular activation of each type of T cell. T-cell activation requires presentation of antigens in the context of a specific HLA antigen. Helper T cells require class II HLA antigens; cytotoxic T cells require class I HLA antigens. T-cell activation also involves IL-1, produced by macrophages, and IL-2, produced by T cells.

Natural killer cells

Somewhat resembling T cells, natural killer (NK) cells are a discrete population of large lymphocytes. NK cells recognize surface changes on body cells infected with a virus; they then bind to and often kill the infected cells.

Macrophages

Important cells of the reticuloendothelial system, macrophages influence both immune and inflammatory responses. They may circulate in the blood or collect in tissues and organs, such as the liver, spleen, lungs, and connective tissue. Macrophage precursors circulate in the blood. When they collect in tissues and organs, they differentiate into macrophages with varying characteristics. Unlike B and T lymphocytes, macrophages lack surface receptors for specific antigens; instead, they have receptors for the C region of the heavy chain (Fc region) of immunoglobulin, for fragments of the third component of complement (C3), and for nonimmunologic factors such as carbohydrate molecules.

Macrophages ingest and process antigen and then deposit it on their own surfaces in association with HLA antigen. T lymphocytes become activated upon recognizing this complex. Macrophages also function in the inflammatory response by producing IL-1, which generates fever, and by synthesizing complement proteins and other mediators that produce phagocytic, microbicidal, and tumoricidal effects.

Cytokines

Communication between cells involves cytokines, which are low-molecular-weight proteins. Their purpose is to induce or regulate a variety of immune or inflammatory responses.

However, disorders may occur if cytokine production or regulation is impaired. Cytokines are categorized as follows:

• Colony-stimulating factors function primarily as hematopoietic growth factors, guiding the division and differentiation of bone marrow stem cells. They also influence the functioning of mature lymphocytes, monocytes, macrophages, and neutrophils.

• Interferons act very early to limit the spread of viral infections. They also inhibit tumor growth. Mainly, they determine how well tissue cells interact with cytotoxic cells and lymphocytes.

• Interleukins are a large group of cytokines. Those produced by T lymphocytes are called lymphokines. Those produced by mononuclear phagocytes are called monokines. They have a variety of effects, but most direct other cells to divide and differentiate.

• Tumor necrosis factors are thought to play an important role in mediating inflammation and cytotoxic reactions (along with IL-1, IL-6, and IL-8).

• Transforming growth factor demonstrates both inflammatory and anti-inflammatory effects. It is believed to be partially responsible for tissue fibrosis associated with many diseases. It demonstrates immunosuppressive effects on T cells, B cells, and NK cells.

Complement system

The chief humoral effector of the inflammatory response, the complement system consists of more than 20 serum proteins. When activated, these proteins interact in a cascade-like process that has profound biological effects. Complement activation takes place through one of two pathways. In the classical pathway, binding of IgM or IgG and antigen forms antigen-antibody complexes that activate the first component of complement (C1). This, in turn, activates C4, C2, and C3. In the alternate pathway, activating surfaces, such as bacterial membranes, directly amplify spontaneous cleavage of C3. Once C3 is activated in either pathway, activation of the terminal components—C5 to C9—follows.

The major biological effects of complement activation include phagocyte attraction (chemotaxis) and activation, histamine release, viral neutralization, promotion of phagocytosis by opsonization, and lysis of cells and bacteria. Other mediators of inflammation derived from the kinin and co-agulation pathways interact with the complement system.

Polymorpho-nuclear leukocytes

Besides macrophages and complement, other key participants in the inflammatory response are the polymorphonuclear leukocytes—neutrophils, eosinophils, and basophils.

Neutrophils, the most numerous of these cells, derive from bone marrow and increase dramatically in number in response to infection and inflammation. Highly mobile cells, neutrophils are attracted to areas of inflammation (chemotaxis); in fact, they're the primary constituent of pus.

Neutrophils have surface receptors for immunoglobulin and complement fragments and avidly ingest opsonized particles such as bacteria. Ingested organisms are then promptly killed by toxic oxygen metabolites and enzymes such as lysozyme. Unfortunately, neutrophils not only kill invading organisms but may also damage host tissues.

Also derived from bone marrow, eosinophils multiply in allergic disorders and parasitic infestations. Although their phagocytic function isn't entirely clear, evidence suggests that they participate in host defense against parasites. Their products are also involved in allergic disorders.

Two other cells that function in allergic disorders are basophils and mast cells. (Mast cells, however, are not blood cells.) Basophils circulate in peripheral blood, whereas mast cells accumulate in connective tissue, particularly in the lungs, intestines, and skin. Both cells have surface receptors for IgE. When cross-linked by an IgE-antigen complex, they release allergic mediators.

Immune disorders

Because of their complexity, the processes involved in host defense and immune response may malfunction. When the body's defenses are exaggerated, misdirected, or either absent or depressed, the result may be a hypersensitivity disorder, autoimmunity, or immunodeficiency, respectively.

Hypersensitivity disorders

An exaggerated or inappropriate immune response may lead to various hypersensitivity disorders. Such disorders are classified as Type I through Type IV, although some overlap exists. (See *Gell and Coombs classification of hypersensitivity reactions*, pages 10 and 11.)

(Text continues on page 12.)

Gell and Coombs classification of hypersensitivity reactions

In 1962, British immunologists P.G.H. Gell and R.R.A. Coombs classified four ways in which immune system activity causes tissue damage. With some modifications, the system remains applicable today.

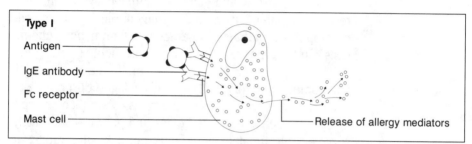

Type I

Antigen —
IgE antibody —
Fc receptor —
Mast cell —
— Release of allergy mediators

REACTIONS	PATHOPHYSIOLOGY	SIGNS AND SYMPTOMS	CLINICAL EXAMPLES
Anaphylactic (immediate, atopic, immunoglobulin E [IgE]–mediated, reaginic)	Binding of antigens to IgE antibodies on mast cell surfaces releases chemical mediators, causing vasodilation, increased capillary permeability, smooth-muscle contraction, and eosinophilia.	*Systemic:* angioedema; hypotension; bronchospasm, GI, or uterine spasm; stridor *Local:* urticaria, pruritus	Extrinsic asthma, seasonal allergic rhinitis, systemic anaphylaxis, reactions to stinging insects, some food and drug reactions, some cases of urticaria, infantile eczema

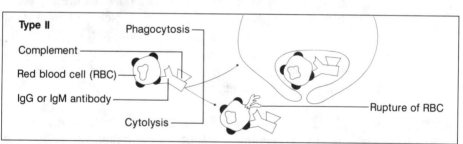

Type II

Phagocytosis —
Complement —
Red blood cell (RBC) —
IgG or IgM antibody —
Cytolysis —
— Rupture of RBC

REACTIONS	PATHOPHYSIOLOGY	SIGNS AND SYMPTOMS	CLINICAL EXAMPLES
Cytotoxic (cytolytic, complement-dependent cytotoxicity)	Binding of IgG or IgM antibody to cellular or exogenous antigens activates the complement cascade, resulting in phagocytosis or cytolysis.	Varies with disease; can include dyspnea, hemoptysis, fever	Goodpasture's syndrome, autoimmune hemolytic anemia, thrombocytopenia, pernicious anemia, hyperacute renal allograft rejection, transfusion reaction, hemolytic disease of the newborn, some drug reactions

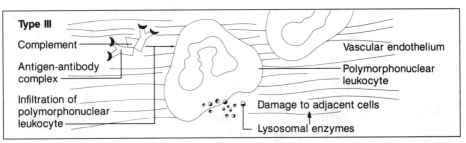

REACTIONS	PATHOPHYSIOLOGY	SIGNS AND SYMPTOMS	CLINICAL EXAMPLES
Immune complex disease	Activation of complement by immune complexes causes infiltration of polymorphonuclear leukocytes and release of lysosomal enzymes and permeability factors, producing an inflammatory reaction.	Urticaria, palpable purpura, adenopathy, joint pain, fever, serum sickness–like syndrome	Serum sickness due to serum, drugs, or viral hepatitis antigen; membranous glomerulonephritis; systemic lupus erythematosus; rheumatoid arthritis; polyarteritis; cryoglobulinemia

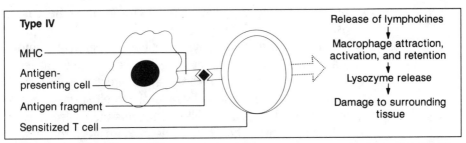

REACTIONS	PATHOPHYSIOLOGY	SIGNS AND SYMPTOMS	CLINICAL EXAMPLES
Delayed (cell-mediated)	An antigen-presenting cell presents antigen to T cells in association with the major histocompatibility complex. The sensitized T cells release lymphokines, which stimulate macrophages; lysozymes are released, and surrounding tissue is damaged.	Varies with disease; can include fever, erythema, and pruritus.	Contact dermatitis, graft-versus-host disease, allograft rejection, granuloma due to intracellular organisms, some drug sensitivities, Hashimoto's thyroiditis, tuberculosis, sarcoidosis

In Type I hypersensitivity (allergic disorders), certain antigens (allergens) in some individuals activate T cells. These T cells induce B-cell production of IgE, which binds to the Fc receptors on the surface of mast cells. When these cells are re-exposed to the same antigen, the antigen binds with the surface IgE, cross-links the Fc receptors, and causes mast cell degranulation with release of various mediators. (Degranulation may also be triggered by complement-derived anaphylatoxins—C3a and C5a—or by certain drugs such as morphine.)

Some of these mediators are preformed, whereas others are newly synthesized upon activation of mast cells. Preformed mediators include heparin, histamine, proteolytic and other enzymes, and chemotactic factors for eosinophils and neutrophils. Newly synthesized mediators include prostaglandins and leukotrienes.

Mast cells also produce a variety of cytokines. The effects of these mediators include smooth-muscle contraction, vasodilation, bronchospasm, edema, increased vascular permeability, mucus secretion, and cellular infiltration by eosinophils and neutrophils. Among classic associated signs and symptoms are hypotension, wheezing, swelling, urticaria, and rhinorrhea.

Examples of Type I hypersensitivity disorders are anaphylaxis, hay fever (allergic rhinitis) and, in some cases, asthma.

In Type II hypersensitivity (antibody-dependent cytotoxicity), antibodies are directed against cell surface antigens. (Alternately, though, antibodies may be directed against small molecules adsorbed to cells or against cell surface receptors, rather than against cell constituents themselves.) Type II hypersensitivity then causes tissue damage through several mechanisms. Binding of antigen and antibody activates complement, which ultimately disrupts cellular membranes. Another mechanism is mediated by various phagocytic cells with receptors for immunoglobulin (Fc region) and complement fragments. These cells envelop and destroy (phagocytose) opsonized targets, such as red blood cells, leukocytes, and platelets. Antibodies against these cells may be visualized by immunofluorescence. Cytotoxic T cells and NK cells also contribute to tissue damage in Type II hypersensitivity.

Examples of Type II hypersensitivity include transfusion reactions, hemolytic disease of the newborn, autoimmune hemolytic anemia, Goodpasture's syndrome, and myasthenia gravis.

In Type III hypersensitivity (immune complex disease), excessive circulating antigen-antibody complexes (immune complexes) result in the deposition of these complexes in tissue—most commonly in the kidneys, joints, skin, and blood vessels. (Normally, immune complexes are effectively cleared by the reticuloendothelial system.) These deposited immune complexes activate the complement cascade, resulting in local inflammation. They also trigger platelet release of vasoactive amines that increase vascular permeability, augmenting deposition of immune complexes in vessel walls.

Type III hypersensitivity may be associated with infections, such as hepatitis B and bacterial endocarditis; cancers, in which a serum sickness–like syndrome may occur; and autoimmune disorders such as lupus erythematosus (LE). This hypersensitivity reaction may also follow drug or serum therapy.

In Type IV hypersensitivity (delayed hypersensitivity), antigen is processed by macrophages and presented to T cells. The sensitized T cells then release lymphokines, which recruit and activate other lymphocytes, monocytes, macrophages, and polymorphonuclear leukocytes. The coagulation, kinin, and complement pathways also contribute to tissue damage in this type of reaction.

Examples of Type IV hypersensitivity include tuberculin reactions, contact hypersensitivity, and sarcoidosis.

Autoimmune disorders

A misdirected immune response characterizes autoimmunity, in which the body's defenses become self-destructive. What causes this abnormal response remains puzzling. Recognition of self through the MHC is known to be of primary importance in an immune response. However, just how an immune response against self is prevented, and which cells are primarily responsible, isn't well understood.

Autoimmunity is believed to result from a combination of factors, including genetic, hormonal, and environmental influences. Many autoimmune disorders are characterized by B-cell hyperactivity, marked by a proliferation of B cells and autoantibodies and by hypergammaglobulinemia. B-cell hyperactivity is probably related to T-cell abnormalities, but the molecular basis of autoimmunity is, at present, poorly understood. Hormonal and genetic factors strongly influence the incidence of autoimmune disorders; for example, LE predominantly affects women of childbearing age, and certain HLA haplotypes are associated with an increased risk of specific autoimmune disorders.

Immunodeficiency

In immunodeficiency, the immune response is absent or depressed, resulting in increased susceptibility to infection. This disorder may be primary or secondary. Primary immunodeficiency reflects a defect involving T cells, B cells, or lymphoid tissues. Secondary immunodeficiency results from an underlying disease or factor that depresses or blocks the immune response. The most common forms of immunodeficiency are caused by viral infection, as in acquired immunodeficiency syndrome, or are iatrogenic in origin.

Immune system evaluation: Health history

A complete evaluation of the immune system usually includes taking a health history, performing a physical examination, and reviewing the results of diagnostic tests. You can identify immune system problems while performing a complete evaluation of the immune system or while investigating a patient complaint.

During the health history, you'll explore the patient's chief complaint and other symptoms, and assess the impact of the illness or complaint on him and his family. You'll also gather information to guide diagnosis and treatment.

Include the patient's family members or close friends when taking the history. They may be able to help you corroborate information you obtain from the patient.

Obtain biographical data, including age, sex, race, and ethnic background. Keep in mind that some immune disorders occur more frequently in certain populations. For example, systemic lupus erythematosus (SLE) appears more often in women than in men.

Chief complaint

Document the chief complaint in the patient's own words. Ask about its onset, duration, frequency, location, setting, and aggravating and alleviating factors. Ask the patient if he has experienced adverse effects from any treatment. If the patient has trouble identifying his signs and symptoms, ask if he has any of these common immunologic complaints: fever, fatigue, joint pain, swollen glands, weight loss, and skin rash. You might ask him, "What made you seek medical care today?"

Illnesses and treatments

Find out if the patient has any disorders or has undergone any procedures that could affect his immune system or influence his recovery. Consider asking such questions as:
• Have you received treatment for cancer or any chronic illness?
• Have you had a recent blood transfusion?
• Have you received radiation therapy or tissue or organ transplants?
• Do you have any allergies?
• Have you had any surgery (such as thymectomy or splenectomy)?
• Have you ever been in an accident or suffered injuries?
• Which prescription or over-the-counter drugs are you taking?

If the patient can't remember which medications he's taking, find out if he brought them to the hospital. If so, examine the labels and contents. Numerous drugs, including corticosteroids, chemotherapeutic agents, and antibiotics, may suppress immune system functioning.

Family history

Because genetic factors have been implicated in many immune disorders, you need to take a thorough family history. Ask if any immediate relatives, such as parents, siblings, and children, have cancer or a chronic disease. If an immediate relative has an immune disorder, inquire about the patient's grandparents, aunts, and uncles.

Lifestyle factors

Review the patient's dietary habits and cultural and social background. Consider the following questions:
• Does his diet include appropriate amounts of protein, calories, and vitamins?
• Is he suffering from anorexia or weight loss?
• Which restrictions and supplements does his diet include?
• Does he react to certain foods? If so, find out which foods and ask him to describe his reactions.
• How would he describe his family and social life?

• Does he use alcohol or illicit drugs? If the patient drinks alcohol, determine the number of drinks he has daily because this may affect specific immunologic treatments.
• Does his work environment expose him to irritating or toxic materials, radiation, infectious agents, or allergens?

Coping patterns

Evaluate the patient's ability to cope with stress. If he has an immune disorder, evaluate how illness has affected his life. Consider the following questions:
• In the past 2 years, have you experienced any major changes in your life, such as the death of a loved one, divorce, marriage, or the loss of a job or a job change?
• Is your job or home life stressful?
• How has the illness affected your job, your ability to perform activities of daily living, personal relationships, and outside interests?
• Do you feel your coping strategies are helping or hindering your progress?
• Is your family supportive? How do they perceive your illness? If the patient's family doesn't live nearby or if they're not supportive, ask if he has any other support systems.

Use information about the patient's coping patterns to determine his teaching needs. When planning care, take into account his level of knowledge concerning his illness and its management. Also consider his motivation to learn. If the patient isn't ready or willing to accept change, he's unlikely to respond to your teaching.

Immune system evaluation: Physical examination

Your next step is to perform a physical examination, including an assessment of the patient's spleen and lymph nodes. Using a systematic sequence of examination techniques will help ensure that you don't miss important findings. Because immune disorders have systemic effects, be sure to consider related body systems and organs.

Overall appearance

When observing the patient's appearance, look for signs of acute illness, such as profuse perspiration, and of chronic illness, such as emaciation and listlessness. Determine whether the patient's appearance reflects his stated age. Chronic disease and nutritional deficiencies related to immune dysfunction may make a patient appear older than his chronologic age.

• Observe the patient's facial features. Note any edema, grimacing, or lack of expression. Nonpitting edema often accompanies myxedema, a severe hypothyroid state.
• Measure the patient's height and weight. Compare the findings with normal values for the patient's age, sex, and bone structure. Weight loss commonly accompanies many immune disorders.
• Check the patient's posture, movements, and gait for abnormalities that may indicate joint, spinal, or neurologic changes caused by an immune disorder.

Mental status

Evaluate the patient's level of consciousness and mental status. Consider the following questions:
• Is your patient alert? Does he respond appropriately to questions and directions?
• Has his mental status changed? A patient with SLE may experience altered mentation, depression, or psychosis. A patient with acquired immunodeficiency syndrome (AIDS) may demonstrate mental status changes due to human immunodeficiency virus, encephalopathy, or opportunistic diseases affecting the central nervous system.

Save time by combining steps. For example, observe the patient's general appearance and mental status as you take the health history. Then confirm your observations quickly at the beginning of the physical examination.

Vital signs

Measurement of vital signs should include the patient's temperature, pulse rate, respiratory rate and character, and blood pressure. Fever may indicate infection, a common occurrence in patients with immune disorders. Because other signs of infection or inflammation, such as redness, swelling, and drainage, may be absent in the patient with an immune disorder, fever and accompanying chills may be the only warning signs of a problem.

Skin, hair, and nails

Observe the patient's skin for any color changes. Normally, the skin has a slightly rosy undertone, even in dark-skinned patients.
• Notice any pallor, cyanosis, or jaundice. Check for erythema, which may indicate a local inflammation, and for plethora (red, florid complexion).

• Observe for telangiectasia (reddish-blue, linear or starlike lesions on the face and trunk), which may be associated with immune disorders such as scleroderma.

• Evaluate skin integrity. Check for signs of inflammation or infection, such as swelling, heat, or tenderness. Also note other signs of infection, such as poor wound healing, wound drainage, induration, or lesions. Pay close attention to sites of recent invasive procedures, such as venipunctures, bone marrow biopsies, or surgery, for evidence of wound healing.

• Check for rashes and note their distribution. For example, a butterfly-shaped rash over the nose and cheeks may indicate SLE.

• Note any palpable, painless, purplish lesions that may indicate Kaposi's sarcoma, an opportunistic cancer common in patients with AIDS.

• Palpate for nodules, especially around joints. You may be able to detect subcutaneous nodules in patients with rheumatoid arthritis (RA).

• Observe hair texture and distribution, noting any alopecia on the arms, legs, or head. Patchy alopecia in these areas and broken hairs above the hairline (lupus hairs) occur with SLE.

• Inspect the color and texture of the patient's nails, which should appear pink, smooth, and slightly convex. Longitudinal striations can indicate anemia. Onycholysis (nail separation from the nail bed) may result from thyroiditis.

Head and neck

To assess the patient's head and neck, take the following steps:

• Test the patient's eye muscle strength using the six cardinal positions of gaze and the convergence tests. Remember that ocular muscle weakness may accompany disorders such as Graves' disease.

• Inspect the external portion of the eyes. Note any periorbital edema, which may accompany glomerulonephritis or other renal disease, hypothyroidism (which may occur in patients with Hashimoto's thyroiditis), or allergic reactions. Observe the eyelids for signs of infection or inflammation. Eyelid drooping commonly occurs in patients with myasthenia gravis.

• Inspect the color of the patient's conjunctivae (normally pink) and sclerae (normally white). Conjunctival pallor may accompany anemia. Erythema may signify conjunctivitis, which accompanies allergic reactions and may be seen in patients with AIDS.

• Examine the fundus with an ophthalmoscope. The retina should be light yellow to orange, and the background should be free of exudate, hemorrhages, and aneurysms. Your ophthalmoscopic examination may also reveal hemorrhage or infiltration with vasculitis.

• Inspect the oral mucous membranes. They should be pink, moist, smooth, and without lesions. Fluffy white patches scattered throughout the mouth may indicate candidiasis, a fungal infection. Lacy white plaques on the buccal mucosa may be caused by hairy leukoplakia. Also look for fluid-filled vesicles on any part of the oral mucosa, which may indicate herpes simplex. Such lesions may occur in patients with immunosuppressive disorders or in those who receive chemotherapy.

• Observe the gums. They should be pink, moist, and slightly irregular with no spongy or edematous areas. Gingival swelling, redness, oozing, bleeding, or ulcerations can signal bleeding disorders.

• Inspect the tongue. It should be pink and slightly rough, and fit comfortably into the floor of the mouth. The tongue may appear enlarged in thyroiditis and may lack papillae in pernicious anemia.

• Inspect the neck for an enlarged thyroid gland. Palpate the thyroid gland, noting its size, shape, and consistency. Certain autoimmune disorders, such as Graves' disease and Hashimoto's thyroiditis, can result in diffuse thyroid enlargement.

Lymph nodes

Use inspection and palpation to assess the patient's superficial lymph nodes, starting with nodes in the head and neck. First inspect the visible lymph nodes. Then palpate those that can't be seen. Apply gentle pressure and rotary motion to feel the underlying nodes without obscuring them by pressing them deeper into soft tissue. (See *Palpating the lymph nodes,* pages 20 to 26.)

If palpation reveals nodal enlargement or other abnormalities, note the location, size, shape, surface, consistency, symmetry, mobility, color, tenderness, temperature, pulsations, and vascularity of the affected nodes. Although lymph

(Text continues on page 27.)

Palpating the lymph nodes

When evaluating a patient for signs of an immune disorder, you'll need to palpate the superficial lymph nodes of the head and neck and of the axillary, epitrochlear, inguinal, and popliteal areas, using the pads of the index and middle fingers. Normally, lymph nodes aren't palpable, tender, or hot to the touch. However, if superficial lymph nodes are palpable, they should be less than 1" (3 cm) in diameter, firm, oval or round, well defined, mobile, nontender, and nonpulsating.

Head and neck lymph nodes
You can palpate the patient's head and neck lymph nodes best when the patient is sitting.

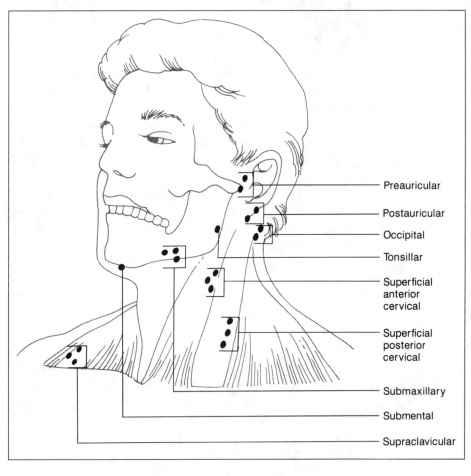

- Preauricular
- Postauricular
- Occipital
- Tonsillar
- Superficial anterior cervical
- Superficial posterior cervical
- Submaxillary
- Submental
- Supraclavicular

Palpating the lymph nodes *(continued)*

To palpate the preauricular lymph nodes, face the patient and place your fingertips over the node site in front of the ear. Continue to sequentially palpate the postauricular lymph nodes located just behind the ear over the mastoid process, the occipital lymph nodes located behind the ear at the base of the skull, and the tonsillar lymph nodes located at the angle of the mandible (as shown).

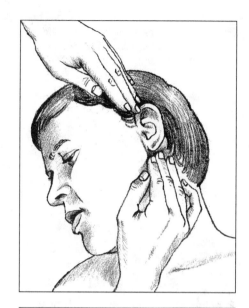

To palpate the submaxillary (submandibular) lymph nodes, flex the patient's head slightly forward or to the side, and place your fingertips over the node site located between the angle of the mandible and the chin. Continue to sequentially palpate the submental lymph nodes located just under the chin and the superficial anterior cervical lymph nodes located over the sternocleidomastoid muscle (as shown).

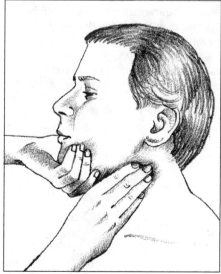

(continued)

Palpating the lymph nodes *(continued)*

To palpate the superficial posterior cervical nodes, place your fingertips along the anterior surface of the trapezius muscle (as shown).

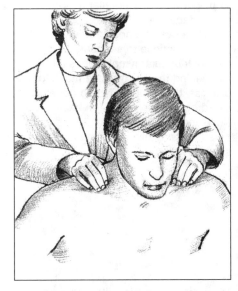

To palpate the supraclavicular nodes, encourage the patient to relax so that the clavicles drop. Flex the head slightly forward. Then hook your left index finger over the clavicle lateral to the sternocleidomastoid muscle (as shown). Rotate your fingers deeply to feel these nodes.

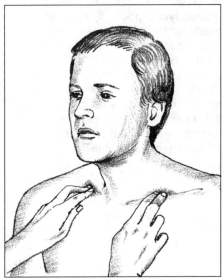

Palpating the lymph nodes *(continued)*

Axillary and epitrochlear lymph nodes

Palpate the axillary and epitrochlear lymph nodes with the patient sitting. You can also palpate the axillary nodes with the patient supine.

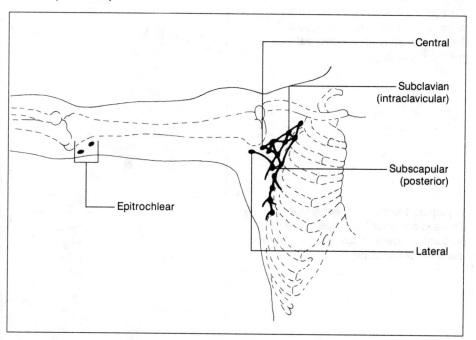

(continued)

Palpating the lymph nodes *(continued)*

To palpate the axillary lymph nodes, have the patient relax. Then reach as high as you can toward the apex of the axilla. Press your fingers in toward the chest wall, and feel for the central lymph nodes (as shown). Then continue to palpate, feeling for the lateral and subscapular lymph nodes. To palpate the subclavian lymph nodes, palpate below the clavicle.

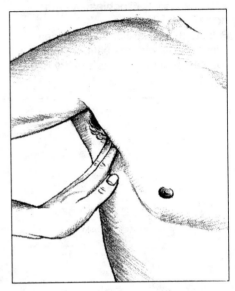

To palpate the epitrochlear lymph nodes, place your fingertips in the depression above and posterior to the medial area of the elbow.

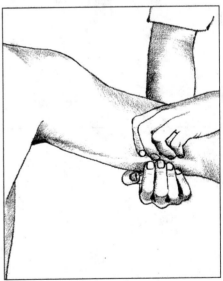

Palpating the lymph nodes *(continued)*

Inguinal and popliteal lymph nodes

Palpate the inguinal and popliteal lymph nodes with the patient in a supine position. You can also palpate the popliteal nodes with the patient sitting or standing.

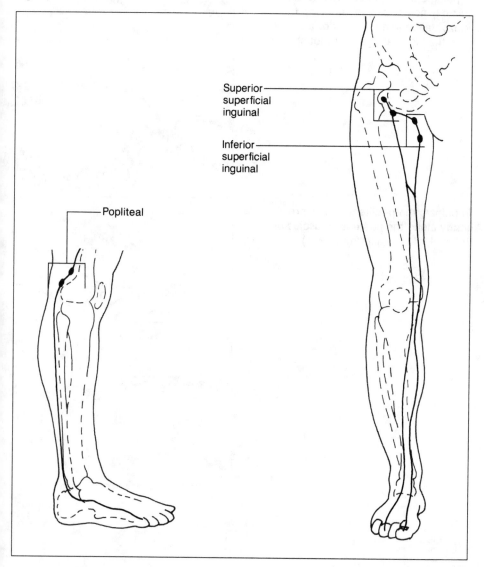

(continued)

Palpating the lymph nodes *(continued)*

To palpate the inferior superficial inguinal lymph nodes, gently press below the junction of the saphenous and femoral veins (as shown).

To palpate the superior superficial inguinal lymph nodes, press along their horizontal course just inferior and parallel to the inguinal ligament (not shown).

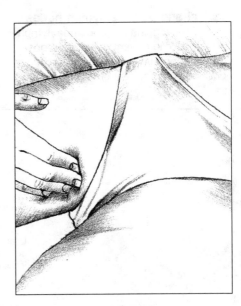

To palpate the popliteal nodes, press gently along the posterior muscles at the back of the knee (as shown).

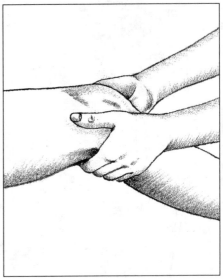

nodes aren't commonly palpable in healthy adults, small, discrete, nontender, mobile nodes may sometimes be palpated successfully.

Enlarged lymph nodes may result either from an increase in the number and size of lymphocytes and reticuloendothelial cells, which normally line the nodes, or from infiltration by cells not normally part of the nodes, as in metastatic cancers. Tender lymph nodes suggest inflammation, whereas hard or fixed nodes suggest cancer. Nodes covered with red-streaked skin suggest acute lymphadenitis. Generalized lymphadenopathy, involving three or more nodal groups, can indicate an autoimmune disorder, such as SLE, or an infectious or neoplastic disorder. In SLE, nodal enlargement may be localized or generalized.

Lungs

Observe the patient's respiratory rate, rhythm, and energy expenditure. Does he exhibit dyspnea, tachypnea, or orthopnea? Note whether he changes position to ease breathing. For instance, during an asthma attack, the patient may sit up and use accessory muscles.

• Percuss the anterior, lateral, and posterior thorax, comparing sides. A dull sound indicates consolidation, which may occur with pneumonia, whereas hyperresonance may indicate trapped air resulting from bronchial asthma.

• Auscultate the lungs to assess for abnormal breath sounds. Wheezing suggests asthma or an allergic response. Crackles may denote a respiratory infection, such as pneumonia, which commonly affects immunocompromised patients. Accompanied by a dry cough, labored breathing, and tachypnea, crackles are a common finding in AIDS patients with *Pneumocystis carinii* pneumonia. Pleural friction rubs may be heard in patients with SLE or RA.

Heart

Auscultate the patient's heart for rate, rhythm, and abnormal heart sounds. Tachycardia or other arrhythmias may accompany anemia, infection, or Graves' disease. An apical systolic murmur may signify severe anemia, which may occur in patients with autoimmune disorders or immunodeficiencies. A pericardial friction rub may be detected in patients with scleroderma, SLE, or RA.

Abdomen

Inspect the patient's abdomen for any lesions, nodules, or scars. Auscultate the abdomen for bowel sounds. In auto-immune disorders that cause diarrhea, bowel sounds increase. In scleroderma and in autoimmune disorders that cause constipation, bowel sounds may decrease. Next, percuss abdominal quadrants to detect tympany or dullness. Tympany usually predominates because of gas in the GI tract. Dullness is normally heard over solid organs. Usually, the liver produces a dull sound over a span of 2½″ to 4¾″ (6 to 12 cm). The area of dullness increases when the liver enlarges.

Also palpate the abdomen to detect enlarged organs and tenderness. You may prefer to alternate percussion with palpation when examining the liver, spleen, and other abdominal areas. Note that hepatomegaly may accompany many immune disorders.

To be palpable, the spleen must be enlarged approximately three times its normal size. In patients with immune disorders, splenic tenderness may result from infections. Percussion of the spleen may reveal splenomegaly, which may result from immune disorders that cause cell overproduction or excessive cell destruction. (See *Percussing and palpating the spleen.*)

Extremities

Evaluate the patient's peripheral circulation by checking for Raynaud's phenomenon (intermittent arteriolar vasospasm in the fingers, toes, ears, or nose), which can produce blanching in the affected area, followed by cyanosis, pallor, and reddening. Next, palpate the peripheral pulses, which should be symmetrical and regular. Weak, irregular pulses may indicate anemia.

To check for musculoskeletal involvement, test the range of motion of the hand, wrist, and knee. Then palpate the joints to assess for swelling, tenderness, and pain. If appropriate, ask the patient to perform such maneuvers as standing up, walking, and bending over.

Diagnostic test results

The results of diagnostic testing complete the objective data base. Along with the health history and physical examination findings, they form a profile of your patient's condition. Blood tests are commonly performed on patients with suspected immune disorders. Other tests include delayed-type

Percussing and palpating the spleen

When assessing the spleen, first use percussion to help estimate its size and to obtain clues about possible enlargement. Then use palpation to detect tenderness and enlargement.

Percussion

Follow these steps to percuss the spleen:

• Percuss the lowest intercostal space in the left anterior axillary line; the percussion notes should be tympanic.

• Ask the patient to take a deep breath, and then percuss this area again. If the spleen is normal in size, the area will remain tympanic. If the tympanic percussion note changes on inspiration to dullness, the spleen is probably enlarged.

• To help estimate spleen size, outline the spleen's edges by percussing in several directions from areas of tympany to areas of dullness.

Palpation

Follow these steps to palpate the spleen:

• Stand on the right side of the supine patient. Reach across her to support the posterior lower left rib cage with your left hand. Then place your right hand below the left costal margin and press inward toward the spleen, as shown below.

• Instruct the patient to take a deep breath. If the spleen is enlarged, you'll feel its rigid border. Note if tenderness is present. Don't overpalpate the spleen; an enlarged spleen may rupture easily.

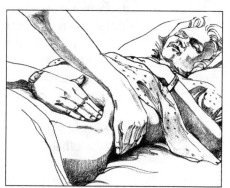

hypersensitivity (DTH) tests, bone marrow aspiration and biopsy, and lymph node biopsy.

Blood tests

The following studies help to determine the effectiveness of the immune system.

Tests of cell counts and activity. These tests require uncoagulated blood. Common anticoagulants used include ethylenediaminetetra-acetic acid, citrate, and heparin. Blood is usually collected in a lavender top tube, using at least a 20G needle to prevent cell damage. To ensure accurate results, tests are performed within a few hours of drawing blood.

• Total white blood cell (WBC) count (reported as number of cells per microliter [μl] or cubic millimeter [mm³] of blood) can provide a general estimate of bone marrow activity.

• The WBC differential provides information regarding the distribution of specific WBCs. This information helps to determine immune function and to assist in the diagnosis of immune or inflammatory disorders. Tests may examine the following WBCs: neutrophils (small phagocytic cells that circulate through the blood in large numbers), monocytes (immature phagocytic cells important in assisting the neutrophils during viral infections), lymphocytes (including T lymphocytes and B lymphocytes), and basophils and eosinophils (small leukocytes that interact with each other). The most commonly measured subsets of lymphocytes are the inducer T cells that express CD4$^+$ and the suppressor T cells that express CD8$^+$. The cluster of differentiation (CD) describes a characteristic cell surface marker. The CD4$^+$ T-cell count and the ratio of CD4$^+$ T cells to CD8$^+$ T cells are important laboratory measurements for monitoring HIV-positive patients.

• Erythrocyte sedimentation rate (ESR) measures the distance that erythrocytes, or red blood cells (RBCs), settle in 1 hour in a tube of 0.9% sodium chloride solution. Erythrocytes normally settle at a specific rate, measured in millimeters (mm). ESR increases with illness and with age.

Serum tests. Important serum tests include immunoglobulin levels, complement assay, radioallergosorbent test (RAST), and the antinuclear antibodies (ANA) test.

• Immunoglobulin levels measure the five different classes of antibodies (immunoglobulin A [IgA], IgD, IgE, IgG, and IgM) formed in response to a specific antigen. The overall concentration of immunoglobulin levels and the distribution of the various types can reveal information about a patient's immune status.

• Complement assay measures levels of complement and its components. Complement is a collective term for a system of serum proteins that control inflammation. Complement assays are based on complement's ability to destroy sensitized RBCs. Reduced levels may indicate that an autoimmune disorder is consuming available complement and using it to form antibody-antigen complexes. Elevated levels may indicate increased complement production. Components of complement are numerically designated as C1 through C9, with C1 having three subcomponents: C1q, C1r, and C1s. (See *Review of laboratory findings in immunologic care,* pages 32 to 34.)

• RAST measures the amount of IgE in the serum directed against a specific antigen. It can determine the severity of specific allergies.

• The ANA test measures the number of antibodies directed at the human cell nucleus. Positive findings from serum diluted to a concentration of 1:16 may indicate an autoimmune disorder, most commonly SLE. (See *Detecting autoantibodies in autoimmune disease,* pages 35 and 36.)

Blood and tissue typing. ABO blood typing, Rh typing, crossmatching, and human leukocyte antigen (HLA) tests help classify a patient's blood for transfusion and other purposes.

• ABO blood typing classifies blood according to the presence of the major antigens A and B on RBC surfaces and according to the serum antibodies anti-A and anti-B. Human RBCs are classified as A, B, AB, or O. ABO blood typing is always required before transfusion to prevent a lethal reaction and before allograft transplantation to help prevent graft rejection.

• Rh typing classifies blood by the presence or absence of the Rh_o (D) antigen on the surface of RBCs. Blood may be typed as Rh-positive, Rh-negative, or Rh_o (D)–positive. Transfusion may take place only if the donor blood is compatible with the recipient blood.

• Crossmatching establishes the compatibility of the donor's and the recipient's blood. This is the best antibody detection test available for preventing lethal transfusion reactions.

• The HLA test identifies antigens on nucleated cells and lymphocytes. Essential to immunity, these antigens determine the degree of histocompatibility between transplant recipients and donors. The HLA test may also aid in establishing paternity.

Other diagnostic tests

Other diagnostic tests include DTH, anergy panel, and biopsies.

• The DTH test assesses general immune function, with the most common DTH being the intradermal purified protein

(Text continues on page 34.)

Review of laboratory findings in immunologic care

Patients with immune disorders generally have detectable increases and decreases of various laboratory test levels. Use the chart below to quickly check the normal adult values and possible causes of increased and decreased values for these tests.

TEST	NORMAL ADULT VALUES	POSSIBLE CAUSES OF INCREASED VALUES	POSSIBLE CAUSES OF DECREASED VALUES
Total white blood cell (WBC) count	• 4,500 to 10,000/μl	• Acute infection • Inflammation • Dehydration • Leukemia	• Chronic infection • Cancer • Bone marrow failure • Immunosuppression secondary to acquired immunodeficiency syndrome (AIDS), chronic cortisol therapy, myelosuppression, antibiotic use, or chemotherapy
Neutrophils (segs)	• 47.6% to 76.8% of total WBC count • 1,950 to 8,400/μl	• Acute infection	• Chemotherapy • Radiation therapy • Neoplastic invasion of bone marrow • Aplastic anemia • Infections, such as viral hepatitis
Lymphocytes	• 16.2% to 43% of total WBC count • 660 to 4,600/μl	• Dehydration • Leukemia	• Acute infection
T cells	• 60.1% to 88.1% of total lymphocyte count • 644 to 2,20l/μl	• Multiple myeloma • Acute lymphocytic leukemia • Occasionally, infectious mononucleosis	• AIDS • Certain congenital T-cell deficiency diseases • B-cell proliferative disorders such as chronic lymphocytic leukemia
CD4$^+$ T cells	• 34% to 67% of total T-cell count • 493 to 1,191 cells/μl	Constitutional in allergy-prone individuals	• Immunosuppression • Cancer • AIDS
CD8$^+$ T cells	• 10% to 49.1% of total T-cell count • 182 to 785 cells/μl	• Viral infection	• Systemic lupus erythematosus (SLE)
CD4$^+$: CD8$^+$ T-cell ratio	• 2:1	• Constitutional in allergy-prone individuals	• Immunosuppression • Cancer • AIDS

Review of laboratory findings in immunologic care *(continued)*

TEST	NORMAL ADULT VALUES	POSSIBLE CAUSES OF INCREASED VALUES	POSSIBLE CAUSES OF DECREASED VALUES
B cells	• 3% to 20.8% of total lymphocyte count • 82 to 392 cells/μl	• Chronic lymphocytic leukemia • Multiple myeloma • Waldenström's macroglobulinemia • DiGeorge syndrome	• Acute lymphocytic leukemia • Certain congenital or acquired immunoglobulin deficiency diseases
Monocytes	• 0.6% to 9.6% of total WBC count • 24 to 960/μl	• Mononucleosis • Viral infection	• Immunosuppression
Basophils	• 0.3% to 2% of total WBC count • 12 to 200/μl	• Inflammation	• Bone marrow failure • Immunosuppression
Eosinophils	• 0.3% to 7% of total WBC count • 12 to 760/μl	• Inflammation • Allergic responses • Helminth infestation	• Bone marrow failure • Immunosuppression
Complement assays	• Total complement: 330 to 730 CH_{50} units	• Obstructive jaundice • Thyroiditis • Acute rheumatic fever • Rheumatoid arthritis • Acute myocardial infarction • Ulcerative colitis • Diabetes mellitus	*Decreased total complement:* • SLE • Acute poststreptococcal glomerulonephritis • Acute serum sickness • Advanced cirrhosis • Multiple myeloma • Rapidly rejecting allografts *C1 esterase inhibitor deficiency:* • Hereditary angioedema *C3 deficiency:* • Recurring pyogenic infections *C4 deficiency:* • SLE
Erthrocyte sedimentation rate	• Men: 15 mm/hour • Women: 20 mm/hour • Children: 10 mm/hour	• Infection • Arteritis • Connective tissue disorders, such as rheumatoid arthritis • Cancer	• Iron deficiency anemia • Sickle cell anemia

(continued)

Review of laboratory findings in immunologic care (continued)

TEST	NORMAL ADULT VALUES	POSSIBLE CAUSES OF INCREASED VALUES	POSSIBLE CAUSES OF DECREASED VALUES
Immunoglobulin levels by immunoelectrophoresis			
Immunoglobulin G (IgG)	• 70% of total immunoglobulins • 500 to 1,600 mg/dl	• Infection • Liver disease • Autoimmune disorders • AIDS	• Agammaglobulinemia • Bone marrow failure • Immunosuppression
IgA	• 15% of total immunoglobulins • 90 to 450 mg/dl	• Liver disease • Exercise • Infection	• Congenital or acquired IgA deficiency • Pregnancy • Protein-wasting disorders • Immunosuppression
IgM	• 10% of total immunoglobulins • 60 to 280 mg/dl	• SLE • Autoimmune disorders • Waldenström's macroglobulinemia • Malaria	• Chronic lymphocytic leukemia • Immunosuppression
IgE	• Less than 1% of total immunoglobulins • 0.01 to 0.04 mg/dl	• Asthma • Allergic conditions	• Immunosuppression
IgD	• Less than 1% of total immunoglobulins • 0.5 to 3 mg/dl	• Chronic infections • Connective tissue disorders	• Immunosuppression

derivative (PPD) test for tuberculosis (TB). In this test, a small amount of *Mycobacterium tuberculosis* is injected intradermally. If the TB bacillus is or has been present, sensitized T cells and antibodies will react with the PPD within 48 hours. However, if a patient is immunocompromised by drugs, disease, or advanced age, no reaction will occur even if TB is present.

• To confirm whether a patient suspected of having TB, but reacting negatively to the PPD test, may actually have TB, an anergy panel is performed. This panel is a series of intradermal injections using derivatives of common antigens. Such antigens include tetanus toxoid, *Candida,* and *Streptococcus.* If none of the intradermal injections causes a positive skin reaction, the patient is considered to have anergy (in-

Detecting autoantibodies in autoimmune disorders

When the immune system produces autoantibodies against the antigenic determinants on and in cells, an autoimmune disorder may result. The chart below lists selected autoimmune disorders, the areas affected, associated antigens and antibodies, and diagnostic tests used to detect autoantibodies.

DISEASE	AFFECTED AREA	ANTIGENS	ANTIBODIES	DIAGNOSTIC TECHNIQUES
Hashimoto's thyroiditis	Thyroid gland	Thyroglobulin, second colloid antigens, cytoplasmic microsomes, cell-surface antigens	Antibodies to thyroglobulin and to microsomal antigens	Radioimmunoassay, hemagglutination, complement fixation, immunofluorescence
Pernicious anemia	Hematopoietic system	Intrinsic factor	Antibodies to gastric parietal cells and vitamin B_{12} binding site of intrinsic factor	Immunofluorescence, radioimmunoassay
Pemphigus vulgaris	Skin	Desmosomes between prickle cells in the epidermis	Antibodies to intercellular substances of the skin and mucous membranes	Immunofluorescence
Myasthenia gravis	Neuromuscular system	Acetylcholine receptors of skeletal and heart muscle	Anti-acetylcholine antibody	Immunoprecipitation, radioimmunoassay
Autoimmune hemolytic anemia	Hematopoietic system	Red blood cells (RBCs)	Anti-RBC antibody	Direct and indirect Coombs' test
Primary biliary cirrhosis	Small bile ducts in liver	Mitochondria	Mitochondrial antibody	Immunofluorescence of mitochondrial-rich cells (kidney biopsy)
Rheumatoid arthritis	Joints, blood vessels, skin, muscles, lymph nodes	Immunoglobin G (IgG)	Antigammaglobulin antibody	Sheep RBC agglutination, latex immunoglobulin agglutination, radioimmunoassay, immunofluorescence, immunodiffusion
Goodpasture's syndrome	Lungs and kidneys	Glomerular and lung basement membranes	Anti-basement membrane antibody	Immunofluorescence of kidney biopsy specimen, radioimmunoassay

(continued)

Detecting autoantibodies in autoimmune disorders *(continued)*

DISEASE	AFFECTED AREA	ANTIGENS	ANTIBODIES	DIAGNOSTIC TECHNIQUES
Systemic lupus erythematosus	Skin, joints, muscles, lungs, heart, kidneys, brain, eyes	Deoxyribonucleic acid (DNA) nucleoproteins, blood cells, clotting factors, IgG, Wassermann antigens	Antinuclear antibody, anti-DNA antibody, anti–ds-DNA antibody, anti–SS-DNA antibody, antiribonucleoprotein antibody, antigammaglobulin antibody, anti-RBC antibody, antilymphocyte antibody, antiplatelet antibody, antineuronal cell antibody, anti-Sm antibody	Counterelectrophoresis, hemagglutination, radioimmunoassay, immunofluorescence, Coombs' test

ability to mount a proper immune defense). Other conditions related to an anergy response include infections, such as influenza, mumps, measles, typhus, and scarlet fever.

• In bone marrow aspiration and biopsy, a specimen of bone marrow, usually from the posterior iliac crest, is taken and used to diagnose various disorders and cancers, such as leukemia, Hodgkin's disease and other lymphomas, granuloma, aplastic or megaloblastic anemia, and thrombocytopenia.

• In lymph node biopsy, lymph node tissue is taken, usually from the supraclavicular region, by needle aspiration or by surgical excision to confirm possible cancer and to evaluate immune function.

Self-test questions

You can quickly review your comprehension of this introductory chapter by answering the following questions. The correct answers to these questions and their rationales appear on pages 149 to 151.

1. As part of the immune system, the thymus participates in:
   a. the maturation of B lymphocytes.
   b. the "education" of T lymphocytes to differentiate self from nonself.
   c. the removal and destruction of circulating antigens.
   d. the production of immunoglobulin and activation of the complement cascade.

2. T-cell antigen recognition requires:
   a. IgD.
   b. IgM.
   c. surface immunoglobulin.
   d. MHC.

3. The function of IgA is to:
   a. defend external body surfaces.
   b. act as the major antibacterial and antiviral antibody.
   c. release vasoactive amines stored in basophils and tissue mast cell granules.
   d. serve as an antigen receptor.

4. One of the most important functions of macrophages is to:
   a. produce IL-1.
   b. generate fever.
   c. synthesize complement proteins.
   d. present antigen to T lymphocytes.

5. The function of interferons is to:
   a. limit the spread of viral infections.
   b. guide the division and differentiation of bone marrow stem cells.
   c. mediate cytotoxic reactions.
   d. immunosuppress T cells, B cells, and natural killer cells.

6. Which complement component must be activated via the classical or alternate pathways before activation of the terminal components of the complement system (C5 to C9)?

    a. C1
    b. C2
    c. C3
    d. C4

7. Which type of hypersensitivity does a transfusion reaction represent?
    a. Type I
    b. Type II
    c. Type III
    d. Type IV

8. Autoimmune disorders are characterized by:
    a. absent or depressed immune responses.
    b. the release of lymphokines by sensitized T cells.
    c. a misdirected immune response.
    d. complement activation.

CHAPTER 2

Allergy

An allergy is characterized by a harmful reaction to extrinsic materials, or allergens. Types of allergies include asthma, allergic rhinitis, atopic dermatitis, anaphylaxis, urticaria and angioedema, and blood transfusion reactions.

Asthma

A reversible lung disease, asthma is characterized by obstruction or narrowing of the airways, which are typically inflamed and hyperresponsive to a variety of stimuli. It may resolve spontaneously or with treatment. Its symptoms range from mild wheezing and dyspnea to life-threatening respiratory failure. Symptoms of bronchial airway obstruction may persist between acute episodes.

Causes

Although this common condition can strike at any age, half of all cases first occur in children under age 10; in this age-group, asthma affects twice as many boys as girls. About one-third of other cases begin between ages 10 and 30; in this age-group, incidence is equal between the sexes. About one-third of all asthmatics have an immediate family member with the disease, and 75% of children with two asthmatic parents also have asthma.

Asthma that results from sensitivity to specific external allergens is known as extrinsic. In cases in which the allergen is not obvious, asthma is referred to as intrinsic. Allergens that cause extrinsic asthma include pollen, animal dander, house dust or mold, kapok or feather pillows, food additives containing sulfites, and any other sensitizing substance. Extrinsic atopic asthma usually begins in childhood and is accompanied by other manifestations of atopy (Type I, or immunoglobulin E [IgE]–mediated allergy) such as eczema and allergic rhinitis. In intrinsic nonatopic asthma, no extrinsic allergen can be identified. Most cases are preceded by a severe respiratory infection. Irritants, emotional stress, fatigue, exposure to noxious fumes, and endocrine, temperature, and humidity changes may aggravate intrinsic asthma attacks. In many asthmatics, intrinsic and extrinsic asthma coexist.

Several drugs and chemicals may provoke an asthmatic attack without using the IgE pathway. Apparently, they trigger release of mast-cell mediators via prostaglandin inhibition. Examples of these substances include aspirin, various nonsteroidal anti-inflammatory drugs (such as indomethacin and mefenamic acid), and tartrazine, a yellow food dye. Exercise may also provoke an asthmatic attack. In exercise-induced asthma, bronchospasm may follow heat and moisture loss in the upper airways.

The allergic response has two phases. When the patient inhales an allergenic substance, sensitized IgE antibodies trigger mast-cell degranulation in the lung interstitium, releasing histamine, cytokines, prostaglandins, thromboxanes, leukotrienes, and eosinophil chemotactic factors. Histamine then attaches to receptor sites in the larger bronchi, causing irritation, inflammation, and edema. The influx of eosinophils, in particular, provides additional inflammatory mediators and contributes to local injury.

Signs and symptoms

An asthma attack may begin dramatically, with simultaneous onset of many severe symptoms, or insidiously, with gradually increasing respiratory distress. It typically includes progressively worsening shortness of breath, cough, wheezing, and chest tightness, or some combination of these symptoms. (See *Determining the severity of asthma.*)

During an acute attack, the cough sounds tight and dry. As the attack subsides, tenacious mucoid sputum is produced (except in young children, who do not expectorate). Characteristic wheezing may be accompanied by coarse rhonchi, but fine crackles are not heard unless associated with a related complication. Between acute attacks, breath sounds may be normal.

The intensity of breath sounds in symptomatic asthma is typically reduced. A prolonged phase of forced expiration is typical of airflow obstruction. Evidence of lung hyperinfla-

Determining the severity of asthma

MILD ASTHMA	MODERATE ASTHMA	SEVERE ASTHMA	RESPIRATORY FAILURE
Signs and symptoms during acute phase			
• Brief wheezing, coughing, dyspnea with activity • Infrequent nocturnal coughing or wheezing • Adequate air exchange • Intermittent, brief (less than 1 hour) wheezing, cough, or dyspnea once or twice a week • Asymptomatic between attacks	• Respiratory distress at rest • Hyperpnea • Marked coughing and wheezing • Air exchange normal or below normal • Exacerbations that may last several days	• Marked respiratory distress • Marked wheezing or absent breath sounds • Pulsus paradoxus greater than 10 mm Hg • Chest wall contractions • Continuous symptoms • Frequent exacerbations	• Severe respiratory distress • Impaired consciousness • Severe wheezing or silent chest • Use of accessory muscles of respiration • Prominent pulsus paradoxus (30 to 50 mm Hg)
Diagnostic test results			
• Forced expiratory volume in 1 second (FEV_1) or peak flow 80% of normal values • pH, normal or increased • Partial pressure of arterial oxygen (PaO_2), normal or decreased • Partial pressure of arterial carbon dioxide ($PaCO_2$), normal or decreased • Chest X-ray normal	• FEV_1 or peak flow 60% to 80% of normal values; may vary 20% to 30% with symptoms • pH, generally elevated • PaO_2, increased • $PaCO_2$, generally decreased • Chest X-ray that shows hyperinflation	• FEV_1 or peak flow less than 60% of normal values; may normally vary 20% to 30% with routine medications and up to 50% with exacerbations • pH, normal or reduced • PaO_2 decreased • $PaCO_2$, normal or increased • Chest X-ray that may show hyperinflation	• FEV_1 or peak flow less than 25% of normal values • pH, decreased • PaO_2 less than 60 mm Hg • $PaCO_2$ greater than or equal to 40 mm Hg
Other assessment findings			
• One attack per week (or none) • Positive response to bronchodilator therapy within 24 hours • No signs of asthma between episodes • No sleep interruption • No hyperventilation • Minimal evidence of airway obstruction • Minimal or no increase in lung volume	• Symptoms occur more than twice a week • Coughing and wheezing between episodes • Diminished exercise tolerance • Possible sleep interruption • Increased lung volume	• Frequent severe attacks • Daily wheezing • Poor exercise tolerance • Frequent sleep interruption • Bronchodilator therapy doesn't completely reverse airway obstruction • Markedly increased lung volume	• Cyanosis • Tachycardia

tion (use of accessory muscles, for example) is particularly common in children. Acute attacks may be accompanied by tachycardia, tachypnea, and diaphoresis. In severe attacks, the patient may be unable to speak more than a few words without pausing for breath. Cyanosis, confusion, and lethargy indicate the onset of respiratory failure.

Diagnosis

Laboratory studies in patients with asthma often show these abnormalities:
• *Pulmonary function studies* reveal signs of airway obstruction (decreased peak expiratory flow rates and forced expiratory volume in 1 second), low-normal or decreased vital capacity, and increased total lung and residual capacity. However, pulmonary function studies may be normal between attacks.
• *Pulse oximetry* may reveal decreased arterial oxygen saturation.
• *Arterial blood gas (ABG) analysis* provides the best indications of an attack's severity. In acute asthma, the partial pressure of arterial oxygen is less than 60 mm Hg, the partial pressure of arterial carbon dioxide ($PaCO_2$) is 40 mm Hg or more and pH is usually decreased.
• *Complete blood count with differential* reveals an increased eosinophil count.
• *Chest X-rays* may also show hyperinflation, with areas of focal atelectasis.

Before initiating tests for asthma, rule out other causes of airway obstruction and wheezing. In children, such causes include cystic fibrosis, tumors of the bronchi or mediastinum, and acute viral bronchitis; in adults, other causes include obstructive pulmonary disease, congestive heart failure, and epiglottitis.

Treatment

In acute asthma, treatment aims to decrease bronchoconstriction, reduce bronchial airway edema, and increase pulmonary ventilation. Treatment after an acute episode includes avoiding or removing precipitating factors, such as environmental allergens or irritants.

If asthma is known to be caused by a particular antigen, it may be treated by desensitizing the patient through a series of injections of limited amounts of the antigen. The aim is to curb the patient's immune response to the antigen.

If asthma results from an infection, antibiotics are prescribed. Drug therapy, which is most effective when begun soon after the onset of signs and symptoms, usually includes:

• bronchodilators to decrease bronchoconstriction. Commonly used bronchodilators include the methylxanthines (theophylline and aminophylline) and the beta$_2$-adrenergic agonists (albuterol and terbutaline).

• corticosteroids (hydrocortisone sodium succinate, prednisone, methylprednisolone, and beclomethasone) for their anti-inflammatory and immunosuppressive effects, which decrease inflammation and edema of the airways.

• cromolyn and nedocromil to help prevent the release of the chemical mediators (histamine and leukotrienes) that cause bronchoconstriction.

• anticholinergic bronchodilators, such as ipratropium, which blocks acetylcholine, another chemical mediator.

Managing asthma attacks

For the most part, medical treatment of asthma must be tailored to each patient. However, the following treatments are generally used:

• *Chronic mild asthma.* A beta$_2$-adrenergic agonist by metered-dose inhaler is used (alone or with cromolyn) before exercise and exposure to an allergen or other stimuli to prevent symptoms. The beta$_2$-adrenergic agonist is used every 3 to 4 hours if symptoms occur.

• *Chronic moderate asthma.* Initially, an inhalation beta-adrenergic bronchodilator and an inhalation corticosteroid or cromolyn are prescribed. If symptoms persist, inhaled corticosteroid dosage may be increased, and sustained-release theophylline or an oral beta$_2$-adrenergic agonist (or both) may be added. Short courses of oral corticosteroids may also be used.

• *Chronic severe asthma.* Initially, around-the-clock oral bronchodilator therapy with a long-acting theophylline or a beta$_2$-adrenergic agonist may be required, supplemented with an inhaled beta$_2$-adrenergic agonist and an inhaled corticosteroid with or without cromolyn. An oral corticosteroid, such as prednisone, may be added in acute exacerbations.

• *Acute asthma attack.* Acute attacks that don't respond to self-treatment may require hospital care, beta$_2$-adrenergic agonists given by inhalation or S.C. (in three doses over 60 to 90 minutes) and, possibly, oxygen for hypoxemia. If the patient responds poorly, systemic corticosteroids and, possibly, S.C. epinephrine may help. Beta$_2$-adrenergic agonist inhalation continues hourly. I.V. aminophylline may be added to the regimen and I.V. fluid therapy begun. Patients who don't respond to this treatment—those with continued airway obstruction and increasing respiratory difficulty—are at risk for status asthmaticus and may require mechanical ventilation.

Managing status asthmaticus

Treatment of this medical emergency consists of aggressive drug therapy: a beta$_2$-adrenergic agonist by nebulizer every 30 to 60 minutes, possibly supplemented with S.C. epinephrine, I.V. corticosteroids, I.V. aminophylline, oxygen administration, I.V. fluid therapy, and intubation and mechanical ventilation for hypercapnic respiratory failure (if PaCO$_2$ is 40 mm Hg or more).

Special considerations

The guidelines you'll follow in caring for an asthmatic patient differ depending on whether your patient is experiencing an acute asthmatic attack or needs long-term care. Some considerations apply to all asthmatic patients.

During an acute asthmatic attack

• First assess the severity of asthma.
• Administer treatment and assess the patient's response.
• Place the patient in high Fowler's position. Encourage pursed-lip and diaphragmatic breathing. Help him to relax.
• Monitor the patient's vital signs. Keep in mind that developing or increasing tachypnea may indicate worsening asthma and that tachycardia may indicate worsening asthma or drug toxicity. Blood pressure readings may reveal pulsus paradoxus, indicating severe asthma. Hypertension may indicate asthma-related hypoxemia.
• Administer humidified oxygen by nasal cannula at 2 liters/minute to ease breathing and to increase arterial oxygen saturation (SaO$_2$). Later, adjust oxygen according to the patient's vital signs and ABG levels.
• Anticipate intubation and mechanical ventilation if the patient fails to maintain adequate oxygenation.
• Monitor serum theophylline levels to ensure that they are in the therapeutic range. Observe your patient for signs of theophylline toxicity (vomiting, diarrhea, and headache) as

well as for signs of subtherapeutic dosage (respiratory distress and increased wheezing).
• Observe the frequency and severity of your patient's cough, and note whether it's productive. Then auscultate his lungs, noting adventitious or absent breath sounds. If his cough isn't productive and rhonchi are present, teach him effective coughing techniques. If the patient can tolerate postural drainage and chest percussion, perform these procedures to clear secretions. Suction an intubated patient as needed.
• Treat dehydration with I.V. fluids until the patient can tolerate oral fluids, which will help loosen secretions.
• If conservative treatment fails to improve the airway obstruction, anticipate bronchoscopy or bronchial lavage when the area of collapse is a lobe or larger.

Long-term care
• Monitor the patient's respiratory status to detect baseline changes, to assess response to treatment, and to prevent or detect complications.
• Auscultate the lungs frequently, noting the degree of wheezing and quality of air movement.
• Review ABG levels, pulmonary function test results, and SaO_2 readings.
• If the patient is taking systemic corticosteroids, observe for complications, such as elevated blood glucose levels and friable skin and bruising.
• Cushingoid effects resulting from long-term use of corticosteroids may be minimized by alternate-day dosage or use of prescribed inhalable corticosteroids.
• If the patient is taking corticosteroids by inhaler, watch for signs of candidal infection in the mouth and pharynx. Using an extender device and rinsing the mouth afterward may prevent this.
• Observe the patient's anxiety level. Keep in mind that measures that reduce hypoxemia and breathlessness should help relieve anxiety.
• Keep the room temperature comfortable and use an air conditioner or a fan in hot, humid weather.
• Control exercise-induced asthma by instructing the patient to use a bronchodilator or cromolyn 30 minutes before exercise. Also instruct him to use pursed-lip breathing while exercising.

For all patients

• Teach the patient and his family to avoid known allergens and irritants.

• Describe prescribed drugs, including their names, dosages, actions, adverse effects, and special instructions.

• Teach the patient how to use a metered-dose inhaler. If he has difficulty using an inhaler, he may need an extender device to optimize drug delivery and lower the risk of candidal infection with orally inhaled corticosteroids.

• If the patient has moderate to severe asthma, explain how to use a peak flowmeter to measure the degree of airway obstruction. Tell him to keep a record of peak flow readings and to bring it to medical appointments. Explain the importance of calling the doctor at once if the peak flow reading drops suddenly. (A drop can signal severe respiratory problems.)

• Tell the patient to notify the doctor if he develops a fever over 100° F (37.8° C), chest pain, shortness of breath without coughing or exercising, or uncontrollable coughing. An uncontrollable asthma attack requires immediate attention.

• Teach the patient diaphragmatic and pursed-lip breathing as well as effective coughing techniques.

• Urge him to drink at least 3 quarts (3 liters) of fluids daily to help loosen secretions and maintain hydration.

Allergic rhinitis

This disorder is a reaction to airborne (inhaled) allergens. Depending on the allergen, the resulting rhinitis and conjunctivitis may be seasonal (hay fever) or occur year-round (perennial allergic rhinitis). Allergic rhinitis is the most common atopic allergic reaction, affecting over 20 million Americans. It's most prevalent in young children and adolescents but can occur in all age-groups.

Causes

Hay fever reflects an immunoglobulin E (IgE)–mediated Type I hypersensitivity response to an environmental antigen (allergen) in a genetically susceptible individual. It's usually induced by wind-borne pollens: in spring by tree pollens (oak, elm, maple, alder, birch, cottonwood); in summer by grass pollens (sheep sorrel, English plantain); and in the fall by weed pollens (ragweed). Occasionally, hay fever is induced by allergy to fungal spores.

In perennial allergic rhinitis, inhaled allergens provoke antigen responses that produce recurring symptoms year-round. The major perennial allergens and irritants are dust mites, feather pillows, mold, cigarette smoke, upholstery, and animal dander. Seasonal pollen allergy may exacerbate symptoms of perennial allergic rhinitis.

Signs and symptoms

In hay fever, the key signs and symptoms are paroxysmal sneezing, profuse watery rhinorrhea, nasal obstruction or congestion, and pruritus of the nose and eyes, usually accompanied by pale, cyanotic, edematous nasal mucosa; red and edematous eyelids and conjunctivae; excessive lacrimation; and headache. Some patients also complain of itching in the throat and malaise.

In perennial allergic rhinitis, conjunctivitis and other extranasal effects are rare, but chronic nasal obstruction is common and often extends to eustachian tube obstruction, particularly in children.

In both types of allergic rhinitis, dark circles may appear under the patient's eyes ("allergic shiners") because of venous congestion in the maxillary sinuses. The severity of signs and symptoms may vary from year to year.

Diagnosis

Microscopic examination of sputum and nasal secretions reveals large numbers of eosinophils. Blood chemistry shows normal or elevated IgE levels. A firm diagnosis rests on the patient's personal and family history of allergies and on physical examination findings during a symptomatic phase. Skin testing, paired with tested responses to environmental stimuli, can pinpoint the responsible allergens when interpreted in light of the patient's history.

To distinguish between allergic rhinitis and other disorders of the nasal mucosa, remember these differences. In chronic vasomotor rhinitis, eye symptoms are absent, rhinorrhea is mucoid, and seasonal variation is absent. In infectious rhinitis (the common cold), the nasal mucosa is beet red; nasal secretions contain polymorphonuclear, not eosinophilic, exudate; and signs and symptoms include fever and sore throat. This condition is not a recurrent seasonal phenomenon. In rhinitis medicamentosa, which results from excessive use of nasal sprays or drops, nasal drainage and mucosal redness and swelling disappear when such medication is withheld. In children, differential diagnosis should rule out a nasal foreign body.

Treatment

Effective treatment aims to control symptoms by eliminating the environmental antigen, if possible, and by drug therapy and immunotherapy. Antihistamines effectively block histamine effects but commonly produce anticholinergic adverse effects (sedation, dry mouth, nausea, dizziness, blurred vision, and nervousness). New antihistamines, such as terfenadine, produce fewer adverse effects and are much less likely to cause sedation. However, cardiac arrhythmias may occur with an overdose.

Inhaled intranasal steroids produce local anti-inflammatory effects with minimal systemic adverse effects. The most commonly used intranasal steroids are flunisolide and beclomethasone. Generally, these drugs aren't effective for acute exacerbations; nasal decongestants and oral antihistamines may be needed instead. Advise the patient to use intranasal steroids regularly, as prescribed, for optimal effectiveness.

Cromolyn sodium may be helpful in preventing allergic rhinitis. However, this drug may take up to 4 weeks to produce a satisfactory effect and must be taken regularly during allergy season.

Long-term management includes immunotherapy, or desensitization with injections of extracted allergens, administered preseasonally, coseasonally, or perennially. Seasonal allergies require particularly close dosage regulation.

Special considerations

• When caring for the patient with allergic rhinitis, monitor his compliance with prescribed drug treatment regimens and note any changes in symptom control or signs of drug misuse.

• Before administering any injections, assess the patient's symptoms. Afterward, watch for adverse reactions, including anaphylaxis and severe localized erythema. Keep epinephrine and emergency resuscitative equipment available.

Observe the patient for 30 minutes after the injection. Tell him to call the doctor if a delayed reaction occurs.

• Advise patients to reduce environmental exposure to airborne allergens by sleeping with the windows closed, by avoiding the countryside during pollination seasons, by using air conditioning to filter allergens and minimize moisture and dust, and by eliminating dust-collecting items, such as wool blankets, deep-pile carpets, and heavy drapes, from the home. Occasionally, in severe and resistant cases, patients may have to consider drastic changes in lifestyle, such as relocation to a pollen-free area either seasonally or year-round. Some patients develop complications, including sinusitis and nasal polyps.

Atopic dermatitis

This chronic skin disorder is characterized by superficial skin inflammation and intense itching. Although atopic dermatitis may appear at any age, it typically begins during infancy or early childhood. It may then subside spontaneously, followed by exacerbations in late childhood, adolescence, or early adulthood. Atopic dermatitis affects approximately 0.7% of the population.

Causes

The cause of atopic dermatitis is still unknown. However, several theories attempt to explain its pathogenesis. One theory suggests an underlying metabolically or biochemically induced skin disorder that's genetically linked to elevated serum immunoglobulin E (IgE) levels; another suggests defective T-cell function.

Exacerbating factors of atopic dermatitis include irritants, infections (commonly caused by *Staphylococcus aureus*), and some allergens. Although no reliable link exists between atopic dermatitis and exposure to inhalant allergens (such as house dust and animal dander), exposure to food allergens (such as soybeans, fish, or nuts) may coincide with flare-ups of atopic dermatitis.

Signs and symptoms	Scratching the skin causes vasoconstriction and intensifies pruritus, resulting in erythematous, weeping lesions. Eventually, the lesions become scaly and lichenified. Usually, they're located in areas of flexion and extension, such as the neck, antecubital fossa, popliteal folds, and behind the ears. Patients with atopic dermatitis are prone to unusually severe viral infections, bacterial and fungal skin infections, ocular complications, and allergic contact dermatitis.
Diagnosis	Typically, the patient has a history of atopy such as asthma, hay fever, or urticaria; his family may have a similar history. Laboratory tests reveal eosinophilia and elevated serum IgE levels.
Treatment	Measures to ease this chronic disorder include meticulous skin care, environmental control of offending allergens, and drug therapy. Because dry skin aggravates itching, frequent application of nonirritating topical lubricants is important, especially after bathing or showering. Minimizing exposure to allergens and irritants, such as wools and harsh detergents, also helps control symptoms.

Drug therapy involves corticosteroids and antipruritics. Active dermatitis responds well to topical corticosteroids such as fluocinolone acetonide and flurandrenolide. These drugs should be applied immediately after bathing for optimal penetration. Oral antihistamines, especially hydroxyzine and the phenothiazine derivatives such as methdilazine and trimeprazine, help control itching. A bedtime dose of antihistamines may reduce scratching during sleep. If secondary infection develops, antibiotics are necessary.

Because this disorder may frustrate the patient and strain family ties, treatment may involve counseling.

Special considerations	• Monitor the patient's compliance with drug therapy.

• Teach the patient when and how to apply topical corticosteroids.
• Emphasize the importance of good personal hygiene.
• Be alert for signs and symptoms of secondary infection; teach the patient how to recognize them as well.
• If the patient's diet is modified to exclude food allergens, monitor his nutritional status.

• Offer support to help the patient and his family cope with this chronic disorder.

Anaphylaxis

A dramatic, acute atopic reaction, anaphylaxis is marked by the sudden onset of rapidly progressive urticaria and respiratory distress. A severe reaction may precipitate vascular collapse, leading to systemic shock and, sometimes, death.

Causes

The source of anaphylactic reactions is ingestion of or other systemic exposure to sensitizing drugs or other substances. Such substances may include serums (usually horse serum), vaccines, allergen extracts, enzymes (L-asparaginase), hormones, penicillin and other antibiotics, sulfonamides, local anesthetics, salicylates, polysaccharides, diagnostic chemicals (sulfobromophthalein, sodium dehydrocholate, and radiographic contrast media), foods (legumes, nuts, berries, seafood, and egg albumin) and sulfite-containing food additives, insect venom (honeybees, wasps, hornets, yellow jackets, fire ants, mosquitoes, and certain spiders), and, rarely, ruptured hydatid cyst.

A common cause of anaphylaxis is penicillin, which induces anaphylaxis in 1 to 4 of every 10,000 patients treated with it. Penicillin is most likely to induce anaphylaxis after parenteral administration or prolonged therapy and in atopic patients with an allergy to other drugs or foods. (See *Using penicillin with caution*, page 52.)

An anaphylactic reaction requires previous sensitization or exposure to the specific antigen, resulting in the production of specific immunoglobulin E (IgE) antibodies by plasma cells. This antibody production takes place in the lymph nodes and is enhanced by helper T cells. IgE antibodies then bind to membrane receptors on mast cells (found throughout connective tissue) and basophils.

On reexposure, the antigen binds to adjacent IgE antibodies or cross-linked IgE receptors, activating a series of cellular reactions that trigger degranulation—the release of

Using penicillin with caution

When administering penicillin or its derivatives, such as ampicillin or carbenicillin, follow these recommendations of the World Health Organization to prevent an allergic response:
• Have an emergency kit available to treat allergic reactions.
• Take a detailed patient history, including penicillin allergy and other allergies. In an infant younger than age 3 months, check for penicillin allergy in the mother.
• Never give penicillin to a patient who has had a previous allergic reaction to it.

• Before giving penicillin to a patient with suspected penicillin allergy, refer the patient for skin and immunologic tests to confirm it.
• Always tell a patient he is going to receive penicillin before he takes the first dose.
• Observe carefully for adverse effects for at least 30 minutes after penicillin administration.
• Be aware that penicillin derivatives also elicit an allergic reaction.

powerful chemical mediators (such as histamine, eosinophil chemotactic factor of anaphylaxis, and platelet activating factor) from mast-cell stores. IgG or IgM enters into the reaction and activates the release of complement fractions.

At the same time, two other chemical mediators, bradykinin and leukotrienes, induce vascular collapse by stimulating contraction of certain groups of smooth muscles and by increasing vascular permeability. In turn, increased vascular permeability leads to decreased peripheral resistance and plasma leakage from the circulation to extravascular tissues (which lowers blood volume, causing hypotension, hypovolemic shock, and cardiac dysfunction).

Signs and symptoms

Anaphylactic reaction produces sudden physical distress within seconds or minutes (although a delayed or persistent reaction may occur for up to 24 hours) after exposure to an allergen. Severity of the reaction is inversely related to the interval between exposure to the allergen and the onset of symptoms.

Usually, the first symptoms include a feeling of impending doom or fright, weakness, sweating, sneezing, shortness of breath, nasal pruritus, urticaria, and angioedema, followed rapidly by symptoms in one or more target organs.

Cardiovascular symptoms include hypotension, shock and, possibly, cardiac dysrhythmias, which, if untreated, may precipitate circulatory collapse. Respiratory symptoms can occur at any site along the respiratory tract and commonly include nasal mucosal edema, profuse watery rhinorrhea, itching, nasal congestion, and sudden sneezing attacks. Edema of the upper respiratory tract, resulting in hypopharyngeal and laryngeal obstruction (hoarseness, stridor, and dyspnea), is an early sign of acute respiratory failure, which can be fatal. GI and genitourinary symptoms include severe stomach cramps, nausea, diarrhea, and urinary urgency and incontinence.

Diagnosis

Anaphylaxis can be diagnosed by the rapid onset of severe respiratory or cardiovascular symptoms after ingestion or injection of a drug, vaccine, diagnostic agent, food or food additive, or after an insect sting. If these symptoms occur without a known allergic stimulus, rule out other possible causes of shock (acute myocardial infarction, status asthmaticus, or congestive heart failure).

Treatment

Anaphylaxis is always an emergency. It requires an *immediate* injection of epinephrine 1:1,000 aqueous solution, 0.1 to 0.5 ml, repeated every 5 to 20 minutes as necessary. (See *Teaching patients how to use an anaphylaxis kit,* pages 54 and 55.)

In the early stages of anaphylaxis, when the patient has not lost consciousness and is normotensive, give epinephrine I.M. or S.C., and help it move into circulation faster by massaging the site of injection. In severe reactions, when the patient has lost consciousness and is hypotensive, give epinephrine I.V.

After the initial emergency, administer other medications as ordered: S.C. epinephrine, longer-acting epinephrine, corticosteroids, and diphenhydramine I.V. for long-term management; and aminophylline I.V. over 10 to 20 minutes for bronchospasm. (*Caution:* Rapid infusion of aminophylline may cause or aggravate severe hypotension.)

Maintain a patent airway. Observe for early signs of laryngeal edema (stridor, hoarseness, and dyspnea), which may necessitate endotracheal tube insertion or a tracheotomy and oxygen therapy.

In case of cardiac arrest, begin cardiopulmonary resuscitation, including closed-chest heart massage, assisted ven-

Teaching patients how to use an anaphylaxis kit

If your patient requires an anaphylaxis kit to use in an emergency, explain that the kit contains everything that he needs to treat an allergic reaction:
• a prefilled syringe containing two doses of epinephrine
• alcohol swabs
• a tourniquet
• antihistamine tablets.

Instruct the patient to notify the doctor immediately if anaphylaxis occurs (or to ask someone else to call him). Then he should use the kit as follows.

Getting ready
• Take the prefilled syringe from the kit and remove the needle cap. Hold the syringe with the needle pointing up. Then push in the plunger until it stops. This will expel any air from the syringe.
• Next, clean about 4″ (10 cm) of the skin on your arm or thigh with an alcohol swab. (If you're right-handed, clean your left arm or thigh. If you're left-handed, clean your right arm or thigh.)

Injecting the epinephrine
• Rotate the plunger one-quarter turn to the right so that it's aligned with the slot. Insert the entire needle—like a dart—into the skin.
• Push down on the plunger until it stops. It will inject 0.3 ml of the drug for an adult or a child over age 12. Withdraw the needle.

(*Note:* The dosage and administration for babies and for children under age 12 must be directed by a doctor.)

Removing the insect's stinger
• Quickly remove the insect's stinger if you can see it. Use a dull object, such

as a fingernail or tweezers, to pull it straight out. Don't pinch, scrape, or squeeze the stinger; this may push it farther into the skin and release more poison. If you can't remove the stinger quickly, stop trying. Go on to the next step.

Applying the tourniquet
• If you were stung on your neck, face, or body, skip this step and go to the next one.
• If you were stung on an arm or a leg, apply the tourniquet between the sting site and your heart. Tighten the tourniquet by pulling the string.
• After 10 minutes, release the tourniquet by pulling on the metal ring.

Taking the antihistamine tablets
• Chew and swallow the antihistamine tablets. (For children age 12 and under, follow the dosage and administration directions supplied by your doctor or provided in the kit.)

Following up
• Next, apply ice packs—if available—to the affected area. Avoid exertion, keep warm, and see a doctor or go to a hospital immediately.
• *Important:* If you don't notice an improvement within 10 minutes, give yourself a second injection by following the directions in your anaphylaxis kit. If your syringe has a preset second dose, don't depress the plunger until you're ready to give the second injection. Proceed as before, following the instructions to inject the epinephrine.

Special instructions
• Keep your kit handy to ensure emergency treatment at all times.

Teaching patients how to use an anaphylaxis kit *(continued)*

• Ask your pharmacist for storage guidelines. Find out whether the kit can be stored in a car's glove compartment or whether you need to keep it in a cooler place.
• Periodically check the epinephrine in the preloaded syringe. A pinkish brown solution needs to be replaced.
• Make a note of the kit's expiration date. Then renew the kit just before that date.
• Dispose of the used needle and syringe safely and properly.

tilation, and the administration of sodium bicarbonate; other therapy is indicated by the patient's clinical response.

Special considerations

• Watch for hypotension and shock, and maintain circulatory volume with volume expanders (plasma, plasma expanders, saline solution, and albumin) as needed. Stabilize blood pressure with the I.V. vasopressors norepinephrine and dopamine. Monitor the patient's blood pressure, central venous pressure, and urine output as a response index.
• To prevent anaphylaxis, teach the patient to avoid exposure to known allergens. In food or drug allergy, the sensitized person must learn to avoid the offending food or drug in all its forms. With allergy to insect stings, he should avoid open fields and wooded areas during the insect season and should carry an anaphylaxis kit (epinephrine, antihistamine, tourniquet) whenever he must go outdoors. In addition, every patient prone to anaphylaxis should wear a medical identification bracelet naming his allergy or allergies.
• If a patient must receive a drug to which he is allergic, prevent a severe reaction by making sure that he receives careful desensitization with gradually increasing doses of the antigen or advance administration of steroids. A person with a known allergic history should receive a drug with a high anaphylactic potential only after cautious pre-testing for sensitivity.
• Closely monitor the patient during testing, and make sure that you have resuscitative equipment and epinephrine available.
• When any patient needs a drug with a high anaphylactic potential (particularly parenteral drugs), make sure that he receives each dose under close medical observation.

• Closely monitor a patient undergoing diagnostic tests, such as excretory urography, cardiac catheterization, and angiography, that use iodine-based radiographic contrast media.

Urticaria and angioedema

Also referred to as hives, urticaria is an episodic, usually self-limited skin reaction characterized by local dermal wheals surrounded by an erythematous flare. Angioedema is a subcutaneous and dermal eruption that produces deeper, larger wheals (usually on the hands, feet, lips, genitals, and eyelids) and a more diffuse swelling of loose subcutaneous tissue. Urticaria and angioedema can occur simultaneously, but angioedema may last longer.

Causes

Urticaria and angioedema are common allergic reactions that may occur in 20% of the general population at some time or other. The causes of these reactions include allergy to drugs, foods, insect stings and, occasionally, inhalant allergens (animal danders, cosmetics) that provoke an immunoglobin E (IgE) response to protein allergens. However, certain drugs may cause urticaria without an IgE response.

When urticaria and angioedema are part of an anaphylactic reaction, they almost always persist long after the systemic response has subsided. This occurs because circulation to the skin is the last to be restored after an allergic reaction, which results in slow histamine reabsorption at the reaction site.

Nonallergic urticaria and angioedema are probably also related to histamine release by some still-unknown mechanism. External physical stimuli, such as cold (usually in young adults), heat, water, or sunlight, may also provoke urticaria and angioedema. Urticaria, which develops after stroking or scratching the skin, is known as dermatographism. It occurs in up to 20% of the population. Such urticaria develops with varying pressure, most often under tight clothing, and is aggravated by scratching.

Several different mechanisms and underlying disorders may provoke urticaria and angioedema: These include IgE-induced release of mediators from cutaneous mast cells; binding of IgG or IgM to antigen, resulting in complement activation; and disorders such as localized or secondary infection (respiratory infection), neoplastic disease (Hodgkin's disease), connective tissue diseases (systemic lupus erythematosus), collagen vascular disease, and psychogenic disease.

Signs and symptoms

The characteristic features of urticaria are distinct, raised, evanescent dermal wheals surrounded by an erythematous flare. These lesions may vary in size. In cholinergic urticaria, the wheals may be tiny and blanched, surrounded by erythematous flares.

Angioedema characteristically produces nonpitted swelling of deep subcutaneous tissue, usually on the eyelids, lips, genitalia, and mucous membranes. These swellings don't usually itch but may burn and tingle.

Diagnosis

An accurate patient history can help determine the cause of hives. Such a history should include:
• drug use, including over-the-counter preparations (vitamins, aspirin, antacids)
• frequently ingested foods (strawberries, milk products, fish)
• environmental influences (pets, carpet, clothing, soap, inhalants, cosmetics, hair dye, insect bites and stings).

Diagnosis also requires a physical examination to rule out similar conditions, and a complete blood count, urinalysis, erythrocyte sedimentation rate, and chest X-ray to rule out inflammatory infections. Skin testing, an elimination diet, and a food diary (noting the time, amount, and circumstances of food consumption) can pinpoint provoking allergens. The food diary may also suggest other allergies. For instance, a patient allergic to fish may also be allergic to iodine contrast media.

Recurrent angioedema without urticaria, along with a familial history, points to hereditary angioedema. (See *Hereditary angioedema,* page 58.) Decreased serum levels of fourth component of complement (C4) and C1 esterase inhibitor confirm this diagnosis.

Hereditary angioedema

A nonallergenic type of angioedema, hereditary angioedema results from an autosomal dominant trait—a hereditary deficiency of an alpha globulin, the normal inhibitor of C1 esterase (a component of the complement system). This deficiency allows uninhibited C1 esterase release, resulting in the vascular changes common to angioedema.

The clinical effects of hereditary angioedema usually appear in childhood with recurrent episodes of subcutaneous or submucosal edema at irregular intervals of weeks, months, or years, often following trauma or stress. Hereditary angioedema is unifocal, without urticarial pruritus but associated with recurrent edema of the skin and mucosa (especially of the GI and respiratory tracts). GI tract involvement may cause nausea, vomiting, and severe abdominal pain. Laryngeal angioedema may cause fatal airway obstruction.

Treatment for acute hereditary angioedema may require androgens such as danazol. Tracheotomy may be necessary to relieve airway obstruction resulting from laryngeal angioedema.

Treatment

Treatment aims to prevent or limit contact with triggering factors or to desensitize the patient to them and to relieve symptoms. Once the stimulus has been removed, urticaria usually subsides in a few days—except for drug reactions, which may persist as long as the drug is in the bloodstream.

Special considerations

• During desensitization, intradermally inject progressively larger doses of specific antigens (determined by skin testing).
• Hydroxyzine or another antihistamine can ease itching and swelling but may cause drowsiness.
• Corticosteroid therapy may be necessary for some patients.

Blood transfusion reaction

Mediated by immune or nonimmune factors, a blood transfusion reaction accompanies or follows I.V. administration of blood components. Its severity varies from mild (fever and chills) to severe (acute renal failure or complete vascular collapse and death), depending on the amount of blood transfused, the type of reaction, and the patient's general health.

Understanding the Rh system

The Rh system contains more than 30 antibodies and antigens. About 85% of the world's population has Rh-positive blood, which means that their red blood cells carry the D or Rh antigen. The remaining 15% are Rh-negative and do not carry this antigen.

lytic reaction. For example, an Rh-negative mother who delivers an Rh-positive baby is sensitized by the baby's Rh-positive blood. During her next Rh-positive pregnancy, her sensitized blood would cause a hemolytic reaction in fetal circulation.

Effects of sensitization

When an Rh-negative person receives Rh-positive blood for the first time, he becomes sensitized to the D antigen but shows no immediate reaction to it. If he receives Rh-positive blood a second time, he then develops a massive hemo-

Preventing sensitization

To prevent formation of antibodies against Rh-positive blood, the Rh-negative mother should receive Rh$_o$(D) immune globulin (human) I.M. within 72 hours after delivering an Rh-positive baby.

Causes

Hemolytic reactions follow transfusion of mismatched blood. Transfusion with serologically incompatible blood triggers the most serious reaction, marked by intravascular agglutination of red blood cells (RBCs). The recipient's antibodies (immunoglobulin G [IgG] or IgM) attach to the donated RBCs, leading to clumping and destruction of the recipient's RBCs and, possibly, the development of disseminated intravascular coagulation (DIC) and other serious effects.

Transfusion with Rh-incompatible blood triggers a less serious reaction within several days to 2 weeks. Rh reactions are most likely in women sensitized to RBC antigens by a previous pregnancy or by unknown factors (bacterial or viral infection) and in persons who have received more than five transfusions. (See *Understanding the Rh system*.)

Allergic reactions are fairly common but only occasionally serious. In this type of reaction, transfused soluble antigens react with surface IgE molecules on mast cells and basophils, causing degranulation and release of allergic mediators. Antibodies against IgA in an IgA-deficient recipient can also trigger a severe allergic reaction (anaphylaxis).

Febrile nonhemolytic reactions, the most common type of reaction, apparently develop when cytotoxic or agglutinating antibodies in the recipient's plasma attack antigens on transfused lymphocytes, granulocytes, or plasma cells.

Although fairly uncommon, bacterial contamination of donor blood can occur during donor phlebotomy. Offending organisms are usually gram-negative, especially *Pseudomonas* species, *Citrobacter freundii,* and *Escherichia coli.*

Contamination of donor blood with viruses such as hepatitis, cytomegalovirus, and malaria is also a possibility.

Signs and symptoms

Immediate effects of a hemolytic transfusion reaction develop within a few minutes or hours after the start of transfusion and may include chills, fever, urticaria, tachycardia, dyspnea, nausea, vomiting, tightness in the chest, chest and back pain, hypotension, bronchospasm, angioedema, and signs and symptoms of anaphylaxis, shock, pulmonary edema, and congestive heart failure. In a surgical patient under anesthesia, these symptoms are masked, but blood oozes from mucous membranes or the incision site. Delayed hemolytic reactions can occur up to several weeks after transfusion, causing fever, an unexpected fall in serum hemoglobin level, and jaundice.

Allergic reactions are typically afebrile with urticaria and angioedema, possibly progressing to cough, respiratory distress, nausea and vomiting, diarrhea, abdominal cramps, vascular instability, shock, and coma. The hallmark of a febrile nonhemolytic reaction is a mild to severe fever at the start of the transfusion or within 2 hours after its completion.

Bacterial contamination causes high fever, nausea and vomiting, diarrhea, abdominal cramps and, possibly, shock. Symptoms of viral contamination may not appear for several weeks after the transfusion.

Diagnosis

Confirming a hemolytic transfusion reaction requires proof of blood incompatibility and evidence of hemolysis, such as hemoglobinuria, anti-A or anti-B antibodies in the serum, low serum hemoglobin, and elevated bilirubin levels. When you suspect such a reaction, have the patient's blood retyped and crossmatched with the donor's blood. After a hemolytic transfusion reaction, laboratory test results will show increased levels of indirect bilirubin, decreased haptoglobin, increased serum hemoglobin, and hemoglobin in the patient's urine. As the reaction progresses, tests may show signs of DIC (thrombocytopenia, increased prothrombin time, decreased fibrinogen level) and acute tubular necrosis (increased serum blood urea nitrogen and creatinine levels).

A blood culture to isolate the causative organism should be done when bacterial contamination is suspected.

Treatment

At the first sign of a hemolytic reaction, *stop the transfusion immediately.* Depending on the nature of the patient's reaction, perform the following:
• Monitor vital signs every 15 to 30 minutes, watching for signs of shock.
• Maintain a patent I.V. line with 0.9% sodium chloride solution, and insert an indwelling urinary catheter; monitor the patient's intake and output.
• Cover the patient with blankets to relieve chills, and explain to the patient what is happening.
• Deliver supplemental oxygen at low flow rates through a nasal cannula or hand-held resuscitation bag.
• Administer an I.V. antihypotensive drug and 0.9% sodium chloride solution to combat shock, epinephrine to treat dyspnea and wheezing, diphenhydramine to combat cellular histamine released from mast cells, corticosteroids to reduce inflammation, and mannitol or furosemide to maintain urinary function. Give parenteral antihistamines and corticosteroids for allergic reactions. (Anaphylaxis may require epinephrine.) Give antipyretics for nonhemolytic febrile reactions; I.V. antibiotics for bacterial contamination.

Special considerations

• Document the transfusion reaction on the patient's chart, noting the duration of the transfusion, the amount of blood absorbed, and a description of the reaction and interventions.
• To prevent a hemolytic transfusion reaction: Before giving a blood transfusion, be sure that you know your hospital's policy on blood administration. Then make sure you have the right blood and the right patient. Check and double-check the patient's name, hospital identification number, ABO blood group, and Rh status. If you find even a small discrepancy, don't administer the blood. Notify the blood bank immediately and return the unopened unit.

Self-test questions

You can quickly review your comprehension of the allergic disorders in this chapter by answering the following questions. The correct answers to these questions and their rationales appear on pages 151 to 154.

Case history questions

Eileen Hubbard has suffered for most of her life with seasonal (spring) allergic rhinitis. Her only sibling also has hay fever, and she remembers both her parents experiencing seasonal allergic problems.

1. Allergic rhinitis experienced in the spring most commonly results from wind-borne:
   a. tree pollens.
   b. grass pollens.
   c. weed pollens.
   d. fungal spores.

2. Besides Mrs. Hubbard's symptoms of paroxysmal sneezing, profuse watery rhinorrhea, and nasal congestion, you would expect to find:
   a. beet-red nasal mucosa.
   b. eustachian tube obstruction.
   c. pale, cyanotic, edematous nasal mucosa.
   d. pale, edematous eyelids.

Mrs. Hubbard has used nonprescription antihistamines such as chlorampheniramine to control her symptoms, but she objects to the sedation and dry mouth they cause.

3. To combat local inflammation with minimal adverse effects, you would recommend:
   a. high doses of astemizole.
   b. intranasal beclomethasone.
   c. cromolyn sodium.
   d. desensitization.

Geraldine Mason, age 11, has recently had an acute exacerbation of the atopic dermatitis she experienced in infancy and early childhood.

4. A health history and physical examination reveal pruritus and erythematous, weeping lesions, some of which have become scaly and lichenified. The lesions are located on the:
  a. volar surfaces of the hands and feet.
  b. chest and abdomen.
  c. eyelids and lips.
  d. neck, antecubital fossa, and popliteal folds.

5. To help limit pruritus, treatment will include topical:
  a. drying agents.
  b. antihistamines.
  c. lubricants.
  d. corticosteroids.

Within minutes of the start of a blood transfusion, Sharon Moses becomes dyspneic and complains of chills, chest tightness, and back pain.

6. Your immediate response is to:
  a. slow the transfusion rate.
  b. administer an antipyretic.
  c. administer an antihistamine.
  d. stop the transfusion.

Additional questions

7. The characteristic breath sound of asthma is:
  a. crackles heard over the lung bases.
  b. wheezing.
  c. laryngeal stridor.
  d. rhonchi heard in large airways.

8. In the patient with asthma, the appearance of confusion and lethargy indicates the onset of:
  a. status asthmaticus.
  b. severe asthma.
  c. respiratory failure.
  d. increasing airway obstruction.

9. Anaphylaxis is always an emergency and requires immediate treatment with:
  a. epinephrine.
  b. vasopressors.
  c. corticosteroids.
  d. aminophylline.

10. When a hemolytic transfusion reaction is suspected, the patient's blood is retyped and crossmatched with the donor's blood. In addition, a urine specimen is collected for:
  a. specific gravity.
  b. creatinine clearance.
  c. anti-A or anti-B antibodies.
  d. hemoglobinuria.

CHAPTER 3

Autoimmunity

Marked by an abnormal immune response to oneself, autoimmunity leads to a sequence of tissue reactions and damage that may produce diffuse, systemic signs and symptoms. Among the autoimmune disorders are rheumatoid arthritis, juvenile rheumatoid arthritis, psoriatic arthritis, ankylosing spondylitis, Sjögren's syndrome, lupus erythematosus, Goodpasture's syndrome, Reiter's syndrome, progressive systemic sclerosis, polymyositis and dermatomyositis, and vasculitis.

Rheumatoid arthritis

A chronic, systemic, inflammatory disease, rheumatoid arthritis (RA) primarily attacks peripheral joints and surrounding muscles, tendons, ligaments, and blood vessels. Spontaneous remissions and unpredictable exacerbations mark the course of this potentially crippling disease.

Rheumatoid arthritis usually requires lifelong treatment and, sometimes, surgery. In most patients, the disease follows an intermittent course and allows normal activity, although 10% suffer total disability from severe articular deformity or associated extra-articular symptoms, or both. The prognosis worsens with the development of nodules, vasculitis, and high titers of rheumatoid factor (RF).

Causes

RA occurs worldwide, striking females three times more often than males. Although RA can occur at any age, the peak onset period for women is between ages 30 and 60. It affects more than 6.5 million people in the United States alone.

What causes the chronic inflammation characteristic of RA isn't known, but various theories point to infectious, genetic, and endocrine factors. A current theory postulates that a genetically susceptible individual develops abnormal or altered immunoglobulin G (IgG) antibodies when exposed to an antigen. This altered IgG antibody is not recognized as self, and the individual forms an antibody against it–an antibody known as RF. By aggregating into complexes, RF generates inflammation. Eventually, cartilage damage by inflammation triggers additional immune responses, including activation of complement (C). This, in turn, attracts polymorphonuclear leukocytes and stimulates release of inflammatory mediators, which enhance joint destruction.

Much more is known about the pathogenesis of RA than about its causes. If unarrested, the inflammatory process within the joints occurs in four stages. First, synovitis develops from congestion and edema of the synovial membrane and joint capsule. Formation of pannus–thickened layers of granulation tissue–marks the onset of the second stage. Pannus covers and invades cartilage and eventually destroys the joint capsule and bone. Progression to the third stage is characterized by fibrous ankylosis–fibrous invasion of the pannus and scar formation that occludes the joint space. Bone atrophy and malalignment cause visible deformities and disrupt the articulation of opposing bones, causing muscle atrophy and imbalance and, possibly, partial dislocations or subluxations. In the fourth stage, fibrous tissue calcifies, resulting in bony ankylosis and total immobility.

Signs and symptoms

RA usually develops insidiously and initially produces nonspecific symptoms such as fatigue, malaise, anorexia, persistent low-grade fever, weight loss, lymphadenopathy, and vague articular symptoms. Later, more specific localized articular symptoms develop, frequently in the fingers at the proximal interphalangeal (PIP), metacarpophalangeal (MCP), and metatarsophalangeal joints. These symptoms usually occur bilaterally and symmetrically and may extend to the wrists, elbows, knees, and ankles. The affected joints stiffen after inactivity, especially upon rising in the morning. The fingers may assume a spindle shape from marked edema and congestion in the joints. The joints become tender and painful, at first only when the patient moves them, but eventually even at rest. They often feel hot to the touch. Ultimately, joint function is diminished.

Deformities are common if active disease continues. PIP joints may develop flexion deformities or become hyperextended. MCP joints may swell dorsally, and volar subluxation and stretching of tendons may pull the fingers to the ulnar side ("ulnar drift"). The fingers may become fixed in a characteristic "swan's neck" appearance, or "boutonnière" deformity. The hands appear foreshortened. Carpal tunnel syndrome from synovial pressure on the median nerve causes tingling paresthesia in the fingers.

The most common extra-articular finding is the gradual appearance of rheumatoid nodules – subcutaneous, round or oval, nontender masses – usually on pressure areas such as the elbows. Vasculitis can lead to skin lesions, leg ulcers, and multiple systemic complications. Peripheral neuropathy may produce numbness or tingling in the feet or weakness and loss of sensation in the fingers. Stiff, weak, or painful muscles are common. Other common extra-articular effects include pericarditis, pulmonary nodules or fibrosis, pleuritis, scleritis, and episcleritis.

Another complication is destruction of the odontoid process, part of the second cervical vertebra. Rarely, cord compression may occur, particularly in patients with long-standing deforming RA. Upper motor neuron signs, such as a positive Babinski's sign and muscle weakness, may also develop.

RA can also cause temporomandibular joint disease, which impairs chewing and causes earaches. Other extra-articular findings may include infection, osteoporosis, myositis, cardiopulmonary lesions, lymphadenopathy, and peripheral neuritis.

Diagnosis

Typical clinical features suggest RA, but a firm diagnosis relies on the following laboratory and other test results:

• *X-rays,* in early stages, show bone demineralization and soft-tissue swelling; later, loss of cartilage and narrowing of joint spaces; and finally, cartilage and bone destruction, and erosion, subluxations, and deformities.

• *RF test* is positive in 75% to 80% of patients, as indicated by a titer of 1:160 or higher.

• *Synovial fluid analysis* shows increased volume and turbidity, but decreased viscosity and complement (C3 and C4) levels; white blood cell count often exceeds 10,000/mm^3.

• *Serum protein electrophoresis* may show elevated serum globulin levels.
• *Erythrocyte sedimentation rate* is elevated in 85% to 90% of patients. (It may be useful to monitor response to therapy, because elevation frequently parallels disease activity.)
• *Complete blood count* usually shows moderate anemia and slight leukocytosis.

A C-reactive protein test can help monitor response to therapy.

Treatment

Salicylates, particularly aspirin, are the mainstay of RA therapy because they decrease inflammation and relieve joint pain. Other useful medications include nonsteroidal anti-inflammatory drugs (such as indomethacin, fenoprofen, and ibuprofen), antimalarials (chloroquine and hydroxychloroquine), gold salts, penicillamine, and corticosteroids (prednisone). Immunosuppressives, such as cyclophosphamide and azathioprine, are also therapeutic. (See *Drug therapy for arthritis*.)

Supportive measures include 8 to 10 hours of sleep every night, frequent rest periods between daily activities, and splinting to rest inflamed joints. A physical therapy program including range-of-motion exercises and carefully individualized therapeutic exercises forestalls loss of joint function; application of heat relaxes muscles and relieves pain. Moist heat (hot soaks, paraffin baths, whirlpool) usually works best for patients with chronic disease. Ice packs are effective during acute episodes.

Advanced disease may require synovectomy, joint reconstruction, or total joint arthroplasty. (See *When rheumatoid arthritis necessitates surgery*, page 71.)

Useful surgical procedures in RA include metatarsal head and distal ulnar resectional arthroplasty, insertion of a Silastic prosthesis between MCP and PIP joints, and arthrodesis (joint fusion). Arthrodesis sacrifices joint mobility for stability and relief of pain. Synovectomy (removal of destructive, proliferating synovium, usually in the wrists, knees, and fingers) may halt or delay the course of this disease. Osteotomy (the cutting of bone or excision of a wedge of bone) can realign joint surfaces and redistribute stresses. Tendons may rupture spontaneously, requiring surgical repair. Tendon transfers may prevent deformities or relieve contractures.

Drug therapy for arthritis

The medications presented below are the usual and preferred drugs for treating rheumatoid arthritis. Other drugs that may be prescribed when the disease is resistant to traditional therapy include prednisone, chloroquine, azathioprine, and cyclophosphamide.

DRUG AND ADVERSE EFFECTS	CLINICAL CONSIDERATIONS
Aspirin Prolonged bleeding time; GI disturbances including nausea, dyspepsia, anorexia, ulcers, and hemorrhage; hypersensitivity reactions ranging from urticaria to anaphylaxis; salicylism (mild toxicity: tinnitus, dizziness; moderate toxicity: restlessness, hyperpnea, delirium, marked lethargy; and severe toxicity: coma, seizures, severe hyperpnea)	• Don't use in patients with GI ulcers, bleeding, or hypersensitivity or in neonates. • Give with food, milk, antacid, or a large glass of water to reduce GI adverse effects. • Remember that toxicity can develop rapidly in febrile, dehydrated children. • Monitor salicylate level. • Teach patient to reduce dose, one tablet at a time, if tinnitus occurs. • Teach patient to watch for signs of bleeding, such as bruising, melena, and petechiae.
Fenoprofen, ibuprofen, naproxen, piroxicam, sulindac, and tolmetin Prolonged bleeding time, central nervous system abnormalities (headache, drowsiness, restlessness, dizziness, tremor), GI disturbances including hemorrhage and peptic ulcer, increased blood urea nitrogen and liver enzymes	• Don't use in patients with renal disease, in asthmatics with nasal polyps, or in children. • Use cautiously in GI disorders and cardiac disease or when patient is allergic to other nonsteroidal anti-inflammatory drugs (NSAIDs). • Give with milk or meals to reduce GI adverse effects. • Tell patient that therapeutic effect may be delayed for 2 to 3 weeks. • Monitor kidney, liver, and auditory functions in long-term therapy. Stop drug if abnormalities develop.
Indomethacin Blood dyscrasias; hemolytic, aplastic, and iron deficiency anemias; blurred vision; corneal and retinal damage; hearing loss; tinnitus; GI disturbances, including GI ulcer, hematuria	• Don't use in children under age 14 or in patients with aspirin intolerance or GI disorders. • Severe headache may occur within 1 hour. Stop drug if headache persists. • Tell patient to report any visual changes. Stress the need for regular eye examinations during long-term therapy. • Always give with food or milk. • A single dose at bedtime may alleviate morning stiffness.
Gold (oral and parenteral) Dermatitis, pruritus, rash, stomatitis, nephrotoxicity, blood dyscrasias, and, with oral form, GI distress and diarrhea	• Watch for adverse effects. Observe for nitritoid reaction (flushing, fainting, sweating). • Check urine for blood and albumin before each dose. If positive, withhold drug administration. Stress the need for regular follow-up examinations, including blood and urine testing. • To avoid local nerve irritation, mix drug well and give deep I.M. injection in buttock. • Advise patient not to expect improvement for 3 to 6 months. • Instruct patient to report rash, bruising, bleeding, hematuria, or oral ulcers.

(continued)

Drug therapy for arthritis *(continued)*

DRUG AND ADVERSE EFFECTS	CLINICAL CONSIDERATIONS
Penicillamine Blood dyscrasias, glomerulonephropathy	• Give on empty stomach, before meals, and separately from other drugs or milk. • Tell patient to report fever, sore throat, chills, bruising, or bleeding. • Monitor urine (for protein and blood), liver function, and complete blood count (CBC).
Methotrexate Tubular necrosis, bone marrow depression, leukopenia, thrombocytopenia, pulmonary interstitial infiltrates, hyperuricemia, stomatitis, rash, pruritus, dermatitis, alopecia, diarrhea, dizziness, cirrhosis, and hepatic fibrosis	• Don't give to breast-feeding or pregnant women or to alcoholic patients. • Monitor uric acid levels and CBC. • Monitor intake and output. • Warn patient to report any unusual bleeding (especially GI) or bruising promptly. • Warn patient to avoid alcohol, aspirin, and NSAIDs. • Advise patient to follow prescribed regimen.

Special
considerations

• Assess all joints carefully. Look for deformities, contractures, immobility, and inability to perform activities of daily living.
• Monitor the patient's vital signs, and note weight changes, sensory disturbances, and level of pain. Administer analgesics, as needed, and watch for possible adverse reactions.
• Give meticulous skin care. Check for rheumatoid nodules, as well as pressure ulcers and skin breakdown due to immobility, vascular impairment, corticosteroid treatment, or improper splinting. Use lotion or cleansing oil, not soap, for dry skin.
• Explain all diagnostic tests and procedures. Tell the patient to expect several blood samplings to allow a firm diagnosis and accurate monitoring of therapy.
• Monitor the duration, not the intensity, of morning stiffness, because duration more accurately reflects the severity of the disease. Encourage the patient to take hot showers or baths at bedtime or in the morning to reduce the need for pain medication.
• Apply splints carefully and correctly. Assess for pressure ulcers if the patient is in traction or wearing splints.
• Explain the nature of RA. Make sure that the patient and her family understand that RA is a chronic disease that requires major lifestyle changes. Emphasize that there are no miracle cures, despite claims to the contrary.

When rheumatoid arthritis necessitates surgery

Rheumatoid arthritis (RA) severe enough to necessitate total knee or total hip arthroplasty calls for comprehensive preoperative teaching and postoperative care.

Before surgery
• Explain preoperative and surgical procedures. Show the patient the prosthesis to be used, if available.
• Teach the patient postoperative exercises (such as isometrics), and supervise her practice. Also, teach deep-breathing and coughing exercises to perform after surgery.
• Explain that recovery from total hip or total knee arthroplasty requires frequent range-of-motion exercises of the leg after surgery; recovery from total knee arthroplasty requires frequent leg-lift exercises.
• Show the patient how to use a trapeze to move herself about in bed after surgery, and make sure that she has a fracture bedpan handy.
• Tell the patient what kind of dressings to expect after surgery. After total knee arthroplasty, the patient's knee may be placed in a constant-passive-motion device to increase postoperative mobility and prevent emboli. After total hip arthroplasty, she'll use an abduction pillow between her legs to help keep the hip prosthesis in place.

After surgery
• Closely monitor and record vital signs. Watch for complications, such as steroid crisis and shock in patients receiving steroids. Monitor distal leg pulses often, marking them with a waterproof marker to make them easier to find.

• As soon as the patient awakens after surgery, have her do active dorsiflexion if she can. Supervise isometric exercises every 2 hours. After total hip arthroplasty, keep the head of the patient's bed raised between 30 and 45 degrees.
• Change or reinforce dressings, as needed, using aseptic technique. Check wounds for hematoma, excessive drainage, color changes, or foul odor—all possible signs of hemorrhage or infection. (Wounds on a patient with RA may heal slowly.) Avoid contaminating dressings while helping the patient use the urinal or bedpan.
• Administer blood replacement products, antibiotics, and pain medication as needed. Monitor serum electrolyte, hemoglobin, and hematocrit values.
• Have the patient turn, cough, and perform deep-breathing every 2 hours; then percuss her chest.
• After total knee arthroplasty, keep the patient's leg extended and slightly elevated.
• After total hip arthroplasty, keep the patient's hip in abduction to prevent dislocation. Watch for any inability to rotate the hip or bear weight on it, increased pain, or a leg that appears shorter—all of these signs may indicate dislocation.
• As soon as allowed, help the patient to get out of bed and sit in a chair, keeping her weight on the unaffected side. When she's ready to walk, consult with the physical therapist for walking instruction and aids.

• Encourage a balanced diet, but make sure that the patient understands that special diets won't cure RA. Stress the need for weight control, since obesity adds further stress to joints.

• Urge the patient to perform activities of daily living, such as dressing and feeding herself (supply easy-to-open cartons, lightweight cups, and unpackaged silverware). Allow the patient enough time to calmly perform these tasks.

• Provide emotional support. Remember that the patient with a chronic illness easily becomes depressed, discouraged, and irritable. Encourage the RA patient to discuss her fears concerning dependency, sexuality, body image, and self-esteem. Refer her to an appropriate social services agency as needed.

• Discuss sexual aids: alternative positions, pain medication, and moist heat to increase mobility.

• Before discharge, make sure that the patient knows how and when to take prescribed medications and how to recognize their possible adverse effects.

• Teach the patient how to stand, walk, and sit correctly: upright and erect. Tell her to sit in chairs with high seats and armrests; she'll find it easier to get up from a chair if her knees are lower than her hips.

• If the patient doesn't own a chair with a high seat, recommend putting blocks of wood under the legs of a favorite chair. Suggest an elevated toilet seat.

• Instruct the patient to pace daily activities, resting for 5 to 10 minutes out of each hour and alternating sitting and standing tasks.

• Adequate sleep is important, and so is correct sleeping posture. Advise the patient to sleep on her back on a firm mattress and avoid placing a pillow under her knees, which encourages flexion deformity.

• Teach the patient to avoid putting undue stress on joints and to use the largest joint available for a given task; to support weak or painful joints as much as possible; to avoid positions of flexion and promote positions of extension; to hold objects parallel to the knuckles as briefly as possible; to always use her hands toward the center of her body; and to slide—not lift—objects, whenever possible.

• Enlist the aid of the occupational therapist to teach the patient how to simplify activities and protect arthritic joints. Stress the importance of shoes with proper support.

• Suggest dressing aids—long-handled shoehorn, reacher, elastic shoelaces, zipper-pull, and buttonhook—and helpful household items, such as easy-to-open drawers, a hand-held shower nozzle, handrails, and grab bars. The patient who has trouble maneuvering fingers into gloves should wear mittens. Tell her to dress while in a sitting position as often as possible.
• For more information on coping with RA, refer the patient to the local chapter of the Arthritis Foundation.

Juvenile rheumatoid arthritis

Affecting children under age 16, juvenile rheumatoid arthritis (JRA) is an inflammatory disorder of the connective tissues characterized by joint swelling and pain or tenderness. It may also involve organs such as the skin, heart, lungs, liver, spleen, and eyes, producing extra-articular signs and symptoms. JRA has three major types: systemic (Still's disease or acute febrile type), polyarticular, and pauciarticular.

Depending on the type, this disease can occur as early as age 6 weeks—although rarely before 6 months—with peaks of onset between ages 1 and 3, and 8 and 12. Considered the major chronic rheumatic disorder of childhood, JRA affects an estimated 150,000 to 250,000 children in the United States; overall incidence is twice as high in girls, with variation among the types. Generally, the prognosis for JRA is good, although disabilities can occur.

Causes

Research continues to test several causal theories, such as those linking JRA to genetic factors or to an abnormal immune response. Viral or bacterial (particularly streptococcal) infection, trauma, and emotional stress may be precipitating factors, but their relationship to JRA remains unclear.

Signs and symptoms

Depending on the type of JRA, signs and symptoms vary. Affecting boys and girls almost equally, systemic JRA accounts for approximately 20% to 30% of cases. The affected children may have mild, transient arthritis or frank polyarthritis associated with fever and rash. Joint involvement may not be evident at first, but the child's behavior may clearly suggest joint pain. Such a child may want to constantly sit in a flexed position, may not walk much, or may refuse to walk at all. Young children with JRA are noticeably irritable and listless.

Fever in systemic JRA occurs suddenly and spikes to 103° F (39.4° C) or higher once or twice daily, usually in the late afternoon, then rapidly returns to normal or subnormal. (This "sawtooth," or intermittently spiking, fever pattern helps differentiate JRA from other inflammatory disorders.) When fever spikes, an evanescent rheumatoid rash often appears, consisting of small, pale, or salmon pink macules, most commonly on the trunk and proximal extremities and occasionally on the face, palms, and soles. Massaging or applying heat intensifies this rash, which is usually most conspicuous where the skin has been rubbed or subjected to pressure, such as that from underclothing.

Other signs and symptoms of systemic JRA may include hepatosplenomegaly, lymphadenopathy, pleuritis, pericarditis, myocarditis, and nonspecific abdominal pain.

Polyarticular JRA affects girls three times more often than boys and may be seronegative or seropositive for rheumatoid factor (RF). It involves five or more joints and usually develops insidiously. Most commonly involved joints are the wrists, elbows, knees, ankles, and small joints of the hands and feet. Polyarticular JRA can also affect larger joints, including the temporomandibular joints and those of the cervical spine, hips, and shoulders. These joints become swollen, tender, and stiff. Usually, the arthritis is symmetrical; it may be remittent or indolent. The patient may run a low-grade fever with daily peaks. Listlessness and weight loss can occur, possibly with lymphadenopathy and hepatosplenomegaly. Other signs of polyarticular JRA include subcutaneous nodules on the elbows or heels and noticeable developmental retardation.

Seropositive polyarticular JRA, the more severe type, usually occurs late in childhood and can cause destructive arthritis that mimics adult RA.

Pauciarticular JRA involves few joints (usually no more than four) and most often affects the knees and other large joints. It accounts for 45% of cases. Three major subtypes exist. The first, pauciarticular JRA with chronic iridocyclitis, most commonly strikes girls under age 6 and involves the knees, elbows, ankles, or iris. Inflammation of the iris and ciliary body is often asymptomatic but may produce pain, redness, blurred vision, and photophobia.

The second subtype, pauciarticular JRA with sacroiliitis, strikes boys nine times more frequently than girls. Patients are usually older than age 8 and tend to be HLA-B27–positive. This subtype is characterized by lower extremity arthritis that produces hip, sacroiliac, heel, and foot pain, and Achilles tendinitis. These patients may later develop the sacroiliac and lumbar arthritis characteristic of ankylosing spondylitis. Some also experience acute iritis, but not as frequently as those with the first subtype.

The third subtype includes patients with joint involvement who are antinuclear antibody (ANA) and HLA-B27 negative and do not develop iritis. These patients have a better prognosis than those with the first or second subtype.

Common to all types of JRA is joint stiffness in the morning or after periods of inactivity. Growth disturbances may also occur, resulting in overgrowth or undergrowth adjacent to inflamed joints.

Diagnosis

Persistent joint pain, rash, and fever clearly point to JRA. Laboratory tests, such as those listed below, are useful for ruling out other inflammatory or even malignant diseases that can mimic JRA and for monitoring disease activity and response to therapy:

• *Complete blood count* shows decreased hemoglobin, neutrophilia, and thrombocytosis.

• *Erythrocyte sedimentation rate, C-reactive protein, haptoglobin, immunoglobulins,* and *C3 complement* may be elevated.

• *ANA test* may be positive in patients who have pauciarticular JRA with chronic iridocyclitis.

• *RF* is present in 15% of JRA cases and 85% of rheumatoid arthritis cases.

• *HLA-B27* is positive and may forecast later development of ankylosing spondylitis.

• *Early X-ray* changes include soft-tissue swelling, effusion, and periostitis in affected joints. Later, osteoporosis and accelerated bone growth may appear, followed by subchondral erosions, joint space narrowing, bone destruction, and fusion.

Treatment

Successful management of JRA usually involves administration of nonsteroidal anti-inflammatory drugs (NSAIDs), physical therapy, carefully planned nutrition and exercise, and minor surgery. Both child and parents must be involved in therapy.

Aspirin is the initial drug of choice, with the dosage based on the child's weight. However, other NSAIDs may also be used. If these prove ineffective, gold salts, hydroxychloroquine, and penicillamine may be tried.

Because of adverse effects, steroids are generally reserved for treatment of systemic complications, such as pericarditis or iritis, that are resistant to NSAIDs. Corticosteroids and mydriatic drugs are commonly used for iridocyclitis. Low-dose cytotoxic drug therapy is currently being investigated.

Physical therapy promotes regular exercise to maintain joint mobility and muscle strength, thereby preventing contractures, deformity, and disability. Good posture, gait training, and joint protection are also beneficial. Splints help reduce pain, prevent contractures, and maintain correct joint alignment.

Special considerations

• Parents and health care professionals should encourage the child to be as independent as possible and to develop a positive attitude toward school, social development, and vocational planning.
• Regular slit-lamp examinations help ensure early diagnosis and treatment of iridocyclitis. Children with pauciarticular JRA with chronic iridocyclitis should be checked every 3 months during periods of active disease and every 6 months during remissions.
• Surgery is usually limited to soft-tissue releases to improve joint mobility. Joint replacement is delayed until the child has matured physically and can handle vigorous rehabilitation.

Psoriatic arthritis

A syndrome of rheumatoid-like joint disease, psoriatic arthritis is associated with psoriasis of nearby skin and nails. Although the arthritis component of this syndrome may be clinically indistinguishable from rheumatoid arthritis, the rheumatoid nodules are absent, and serologic tests for rheumatoid factor are negative. Psoriatic arthritis usually is mild, with intermittent flare-ups, but rarely may progress to crippling arthritis mutilans. This disease affects both men and women equally; usually, onset occurs between ages 30 and 35.

Causes

Evidence suggests that predisposition to psoriatic arthritis is hereditary; 20% to 50% of patients are HLA-B27–positive. However, onset is usually precipitated by streptococcal infection or trauma.

Signs and symptoms

Psoriatic lesions usually precede the arthritic component, but once the full syndrome is established, joint and skin lesions recur simultaneously. Arthritis may involve one joint or several joints symmetrically. Spinal involvement occurs in some patients. Peripheral joint involvement is most common in the distal interphalangeal joints of the hands, which have a characteristic sausagelike appearance. Nail changes include pitting, transverse ridging, onycholysis, keratosis, yellowing, and destruction. The patient may experience general malaise, fever, and eye involvement.

Diagnosis

Inflammatory arthritis in a patient with psoriatic skin lesions suggests psoriatic arthritis.

X-rays confirm joint involvement and show:
• erosion of terminal phalangeal tufts
• "whittling" of the distal end of the terminal phalanges
• "pencil-in-cup" deformity of the distal interphalangeal joints
• relative absence of osteoporosis
• sacroiliitis
• atypical spondylitis with syndesmophyte formation, resulting in hyperostosis and paravertebral ossification, which may lead to vertebral fusion.

Typical serum values include negative rheumatoid factor and an elevated sedimentation rate.

Treatment

In mild psoriatic arthritis, treatment is supportive and consists of immobilization through bed rest or splints, isometric exercises, paraffin baths, heat therapy, and aspirin and other nonsteroidal anti-inflammatory drugs. Some patients respond well to low-dose systemic corticosteroids; topical steroids may help control skin lesions. Gold salt and – most commonly – methotrexate therapy are effective in treating both the articular and cutaneous effects of psoriatic arthritis. Antimalarials are contraindicated because these drugs can provoke exfoliative dermatitis.

Special considerations

• Explain the disease and its treatment to the patient and his family.
• Reassure the patient that psoriatic plaques aren't contagious. Avoid showing any revulsion to unsightly psoriatic patches – doing so will only reinforce the patient's fear of rejection.
• Encourage exercise, particularly swimming, to maintain strength and range of motion.
• Teach the patient how to apply skin care products and medications correctly; explain any possible adverse effects.
• Stress the importance of adequate rest and protection of affected joints.
• Encourage regular, moderate exposure to the sun.
• Consider referral to the local Arthritis Foundation chapter for self-help and support groups.

Ankylosing spondylitis

Also called rheumatoid spondylitis or Marie-Strümpell disease, ankylosing spondylitis is a chronic, usually progressive inflammatory disease. It primarily affects the sacroiliac, apophyseal, and costovertebral joints and adjacent soft tissue. Typically, the disease begins in the sacroiliac joints and gradually progresses to the lumbar, thoracic, and cervical regions of the spine. Deterioration of bone and cartilage can lead to fibrous tissue formation and eventual fusion of the spine or peripheral joints. Ankylosing spondylitis may be equally prevalent in both sexes. Progressive disease is well-recognized in men, but diagnosis is often overlooked or missed in women, who tend to have more peripheral joint involvement.

Causes

Recent evidence strongly suggests a familial tendency in ankylosing spondylitis. The presence of histocompatibility antigen HLA-B27 (positive in over 90% of patients with this disease) and circulating immune complexes suggests immunologic activity.

Signs and symptoms

The first indication is intermittent low back pain that's usually most severe in the morning or after a period of inactivity. Other symptoms depend on the disease stage and may include:
• stiffness and limited motion of the lumbar spine
• pain and limited expansion of the chest due to involvement of the costovertebral joints
• peripheral arthritis involving shoulders, hips, and knees
• kyphosis in advanced stages, caused by chronic stooping to relieve symptoms
• hip deformity and associated limited range of motion (ROM)
• tenderness over the site of inflammation
• mild fatigue, fever, anorexia, or loss of weight; occasional iritis; aortic regurgitation and cardiomegaly; upper lobe pulmonary fibrosis (mimics tuberculosis).

These symptoms progress unpredictably, and the disease can go into remission, exacerbation, or arrest at any stage.

Diagnosis

Typical symptoms, familial history, and demonstration of positive HLA-B27 histocompatibility antigen strongly suggest ankylosing spondylitis. However, confirmation requires characteristic X-ray findings:
• blurring of the bony margins of joints in the early stage
• bilateral sacroiliac involvement
• patchy sclerosis with superficial bony erosions
• eventual squaring of vertebral bodies
• "bamboo spine" with complete ankylosis.

Erythrocyte sedimentation rate and alkaline phosphatase and creatinine phosphokinase levels may be slightly elevated. A negative rheumatoid factor helps rule out rheumatoid arthritis, which produces similar symptoms.

Treatment

No treatment reliably stops progression of this disease, so management aims to delay further deformity by good posture, stretching and deep-breathing exercises and, in some patients, braces and lightweight supports. Anti-inflammatory analgesics, such as aspirin, indomethacin, sulfasalazine, and sulindac, control pain and inflammation.

Severe hip involvement usually necessitates surgical hip replacement. Severe spinal involvement may require a spinal wedge osteotomy to separate and reposition the vertebrae. This surgery is performed only on selected patients because of the risk of spinal cord damage and the long convalescence involved.

Special considerations

• Because ankylosing spondylitis can be an extremely painful and crippling disease, your main responsibility is to promote the patient's comfort. When dealing with such a patient, keep in mind that limited ROM makes simple tasks difficult. Offer support and reassurance.
• Administer medications. Apply local heat and provide massage to relieve pain. Assess the patient's mobility and degree of discomfort frequently. Teach and assist with daily exercises, as needed, to maintain strength and function. Stress the importance of maintaining good posture.
• If treatment includes surgery, provide good postoperative care. Because ankylosing spondylitis is a chronic, progressively crippling condition, comprehensive treatment should also reflect counsel from a social worker, home health care nurse, and dietitian.

To minimize deformities

• Advise the patient to avoid any physical activity that places undue stress on his back such as lifting heavy objects.
• Instruct the patient to stand upright; to sit upright in a high, straight chair; and to avoid leaning over a desk.
• Tell the patient to sleep in a prone position on a hard mattress and to avoid using pillows under his neck or knees.
• Warn the patient to avoid prolonged walking, standing, sitting, or driving.

• Encourage the patient to perform regular stretching and deep-breathing exercises and swim regularly, if possible.
• Remind the patient to have his height measured every 3 to 4 months to detect any tendency toward kyphosis.
• Advise the patient to seek vocational counseling if work requires standing or prolonged sitting at a desk.
• Tell the patient to contact the local Arthritis Foundation chapter for a support group.

Sjögren's syndrome

The second most common autoimmune rheumatic disorder after rheumatoid arthritis, Sjögren's syndrome (SS) is characterized by diminished lacrimal and salivary gland secretion (sicca complex). This syndrome occurs mainly in women (90% of patients); mean age of occurrence is age 50. SS may be a primary disorder or associated with connective tissue disorders such as rheumatoid arthritis (RA), scleroderma, systemic lupus erythematosus, and polymyositis. In some patients, the disorder is limited to the exocrine glands (glandular SS); in others, it also involves other organs, such as the lungs and kidneys (extraglandular SS).

Causes

The cause of SS is unknown. Most likely, both genetic and environmental factors contribute to its development. Viral or bacterial infection, or perhaps exposure to pollen, may trigger SS in a genetically susceptible individual. Tissue damage results from infiltration by lymphocytes or from the deposition of immune complexes. Lymphocytic infiltration may be classified as benign, malignant, or pseudolymphoma (nonmalignant, but having tumorlike aggregates of lymphoid cells).

Signs and symptoms

About 50% of patients with SS have confirmed RA and a history of slowly developing sicca complex. However, some seek medical help for rapidly progressive and severe oral and ocular dryness, often accompanied by periodic parotid gland enlargement. Ocular dryness (xerophthalmia) leads to foreign body sensations (gritty, sandy eyes), redness, burning, photosensitivity, eye fatigue, itching, and mucoid discharge. The patient may also complain of a film across her field of vision.

Oral dryness (xerostomia) leads to difficulty swallowing and talking; an abnormal taste or smell sensation, or both; thirst; ulcers of the tongue, buccal mucosa, and lips (especially at the corners of the mouth); and severe dental caries. Dryness of the respiratory tract leads to epistaxis, hoarseness, a chronic nonproductive cough, recurrent otitis media, and increased incidence of respiratory infections.

Other effects of SS may include dyspareunia and pruritus (associated with vaginal dryness), generalized itching, fatigue, recurrent low-grade fever, and arthralgia or myalgia. Lymph node enlargement may be the first sign of malignant lymphoma or pseudolymphoma.

Specific extraglandular findings in SS include interstitial pneumonitis; interstitial nephritis, which results in renal tubular acidosis in 25% of patients; Raynaud's phenomenon (20%); and vasculitis, usually limited to the skin and characterized by palpable purpura on the legs (20%). About 50% of patients show evidence of hypothyroidism related to autoimmune thyroid disease. A few patients develop systemic necrotizing vasculitis, involving the skin, peripheral nerves, and GI tract.

Diagnosis

In SS, diagnosis rests on the detection of two of the following three conditions: xerophthalmia, xerostomia (with salivary gland biopsy showing lymphocytic infiltration), and an associated autoimmune or lymphoproliferative disorder. Diagnosis must rule out other causes of oral and ocular dryness, including sarcoidosis, endocrine disorders, anxiety or depression, and effects of therapy such as radiation to the head and neck. Over 200 commonly used drugs also produce dry mouth as an adverse effect. In patients with salivary gland enlargement and severe lymphoid infiltration, diagnosis must rule out cancer.

Laboratory values include elevated erythrocyte sedimentation rate in most patients, mild anemia and leukopenia in 30% of patients, and hypergammaglobulinemia in 50% of patients. Autoantibodies are also common, including SSA (anti-Ro) and SSB (anti-La), which are antinuclear and antisalivary duct antibodies. From 75% to 90% of patients test positive for rheumatoid factor; 90%, for antinuclear antibodies.

Other tests help support this diagnosis. Schirmer's test and slit-lamp examination with rose bengal dye are used to measure eye involvement. Salivary gland involvement is evaluated by measuring the volume of parotid saliva and by secretory sialography and salivary scintigraphy. Lower lip biopsy shows salivary gland infiltration by lymphocytes.

Treatment

Usually symptomatic, treatment includes conservative measures to relieve ocular or oral dryness. Dry mouth can be relieved by using a methylcellulose swab or spray and by drinking plenty of fluids, especially at mealtime. Meticulous oral hygiene is essential, including regular flossing, brushing, and fluoride treatment at home and frequent dental checkups.

Artificial tears may be instilled as often as every half hour to prevent eye damage (corneal ulcerations, corneal opacifications) from insufficient tear secretions. Some patients may also benefit from instillation of an eye ointment at bedtime, or from twice-daily use of sustained-release hydroxypropyl cellulose capsules. If infection develops, antibiotics should be given immediately; topical steroids should be avoided.

Other treatment measures vary with associated extraglandular findings. Parotid gland enlargement requires local heat and analgesics; pulmonary and renal interstitial disease, corticosteroids; accompanying lymphoma, a combination of chemotherapy, surgery, or radiation.

Special considerations

• Advise the patient to avoid drugs that decrease saliva production, such as atropine derivatives, antihistamines, anticholinergics, and antidepressants.
• If mouth lesions make eating painful, suggest high-protein, high-caloric liquid supplements to prevent malnutrition.
• Instruct the patient to avoid sugar, which contributes to dental caries, and tobacco, alcohol, and spicy, salty, or highly acidic foods, which cause mouth irritation.
• Suggest the use of sunglasses to protect the patient's eyes from dust, wind, and strong light. Moisture chamber spectacles may also be helpful.
• Because dry eyes are more susceptible to infection, advise the patient to keep her face clean and to avoid rubbing her eyes.

• To help relieve respiratory dryness, stress the need to humidify home and work environments. Suggest 0.9% sodium chloride solution drops or aerosolized spray for nasal dryness.
• Advise the patient to avoid prolonged hot showers and baths and to use moisturizing lotions to help protect dry skin. Suggest a water-soluble lubricant to relieve vaginal dryness.
• Refer the patient to her local chapter of the Sjögren's Syndrome Foundation for additional information and support.

Lupus erythematosus

A chronic inflammatory disorder of the connective tissues, lupus erythematosus appears in two forms: systemic lupus erythematosus (SLE), which affects multiple organ systems (as well as the skin), and discoid lupus erythematosus, which affects only the skin. (See *Discoid lupus erythematosus.*) Like rheumatoid arthritis (RA), SLE is characterized by recurring remissions and exacerbations, which are especially common during the spring and summer.

The annual incidence of SLE averages 27.5 cases per 1 million among whites and 75.4 cases per 1 million among blacks. It strikes women 8 times as often as men, increasing to 15 times as often during childbearing years. SLE occurs worldwide but is most prevalent among Asians and blacks. Although the disease can be fatal, the prognosis improves with early detection and treatment. The prognosis remains poor for patients who develop cardiovascular, renal, or neurologic complications or severe bacterial infections.

Causes

The exact cause of SLE remains a mystery, but available evidence points to interrelated immunologic, environmental, hormonal, and genetic factors. Immune dysfunction, in the form of autoimmunity, is thought to be the primary causative mechanism. In autoimmunity, the body produces antibodies against its own cells such as the antinuclear antibody (ANA). The formed antigen-antibody complexes can suppress the body's normal immunity and damage tissues. One

Discoid lupus erythematosus

A form of lupus erythematosus, discoid lupus erythematosus (DLE) is marked by chronic skin eruptions that, if untreated, can lead to scarring and permanent disfigurement. About 1 out of 20 patients with DLE later develops systemic lupus erythematosus (SLE). The exact cause of DLE is unknown, but some evidence suggests an autoimmune defect. An estimated 60% of patients with DLE are women in their late twenties or older. This disease is rare in children.

Signs and symptoms

DLE lesions are raised, red, scaling plaques, with follicular plugging and central atrophy. The raised edges and sunken centers give them a coin-like appearance. Although these lesions can appear anywhere on the body, they usually erupt on the face, scalp, ears, neck, and arms or on any part of the body that's exposed to sunlight. Such lesions can resolve completely or may cause hypopigmentation or hyperpigmentation, atrophy, and scarring. Facial plaques sometimes assume the butterfly pattern characteristic of SLE. Hair tends to become brittle or may fall out in patches.

Diagnostic tests

As a rule, the patient's health history and the appearance of the rash itself are diagnostic markers. The lupus erythematosus cell test is positive in less than 10% of patients. Skin biopsy of lesions reveals immunoglobulins or complement components. SLE must be ruled out.

Treatment

Patients with DLE should avoid prolonged exposure to the sun, fluorescent lighting, or reflected sunlight. They should wear protective clothing, use sunscreen, avoid engaging in outdoor activities during periods of most intense sunlight (between 10 a.m. and 2 p.m.), and report any changes in the lesions. Drug treatment consists of topical, intralesional, or systemic medication, as in SLE.

significant feature in patients with SLE is their ability to produce antibodies against many different tissue components, such as red blood cells (RBCs), neutrophils, platelets, lymphocytes, or almost any organ or tissue in the body.

Certain predisposing factors may make a person susceptible to SLE. Physical or mental stress, streptococcal or viral infections, exposure to sunlight or ultraviolet light, immunization, pregnancy, and abnormal estrogen metabolism may all affect the development of this disease.

SLE also may be triggered or aggravated by treatment with certain drugs—for example, procainamide, hydralazine, anticonvulsants and, less frequently, penicillins, sulfa drugs, and oral contraceptives.

Signs of systemic lupus erythematosus

Diagnosing systemic lupus erythematosus (SLE) is far from easy because SLE often mimics other diseases; symptoms may be vague and vary greatly from patient to patient. For these reasons, the American Rheumatism Association has issued a list of criteria for classification of SLE, to be used primarily for consistency in epidemiologic surveys. Usually, four or more of these symptoms are present at some time during the course of the disease:

• malar rash
• discoid rash
• photosensitivity
• oral or nasopharyngeal ulcerations
• nonerosive arthritis (of two or more peripheral joints)
• pleuritis or pericarditis
• profuse proteinuria (exceeding 0.5 g/day) or excessive cellular casts in the urine
• seizures or psychoses
• hemolytic anemia, leukopenia, lymphopenia, or thrombocytopenia
• positive lupus erythematosus cell, anti-deoxyribonucleic acid, or anti-Smith test or chronic false-positive serologic test for syphilis
• abnormal titer of antinuclear antibody.

Signs and symptoms

The onset of SLE may be acute or insidious and produces no characteristic clinical pattern. However, its symptoms commonly include fever, weight loss, malaise and fatigue, as well as skin rashes and polyarthralgia. (See *Signs of systemic lupus erythematosus*.) SLE may involve every organ system. In 90% of patients, joint involvement is similiar to that seen in RA.

Skin lesions typically manifest as an erythematous rash in areas exposed to light. The classic butterfly rash over the nose and cheeks occurs in fewer than 50% of patients. (See *Butterfly rash.*) Ultraviolet rays often provoke or aggravate skin eruptions. Vasculitis can develop (especially in the digits), possibly leading to infarctive lesions, necrotic leg ulcers, or digital gangrene. Raynaud's phenomenon appears in about 20% of patients. Patchy alopecia and painless ulcers of the mucous membranes are common.

Constitutional symptoms of SLE include aching, malaise, fatigue, low-grade or spiking fever, chills, anorexia, and weight loss. Lymph node enlargement (diffuse or focal, and nontender), abdominal pain, nausea, vomiting, diarrhea, and constipation may occur. Women may experience irregular menstrual periods or amenorrhea during the active phase of SLE.

Butterfly rash

In the classic butterfly rash, lesions appear on the cheeks and the bridge of the nose, creating a characteristic butterfly pattern. The rash may vary in severity from malar erythema to discoid lesions (plaque).

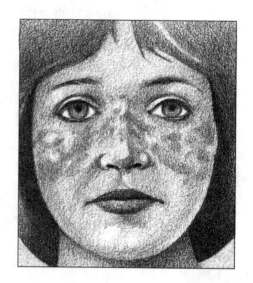

About 50% of SLE patients develop signs of cardiopulmonary abnormalities, such as pleuritis, pericarditis, and dyspnea. Myocarditis, endocarditis, tachycardia, parenchymal infiltrates, and pneumonitis may occur. Renal effects may include hematuria, proteinuria, urine sediment, and cellular casts and may progress to total kidney failure. Urinary tract infections may result from heightened susceptibility to infection. Seizure disorders and mental dysfunction may indicate neurologic damage. Central nervous system (CNS) involvement may produce emotional instability, psychosis, and organic brain syndrome. Headaches, irritability, and depression are common.

Diagnosis

Diagnostic tests in SLE include a complete blood count with differential, which may show anemia and a decreased white blood cell (WBC) count; platelet count, which may be decreased; erythrocyte sedimentation rate, which is often elevated; and serum electrophoresis, which may show hypergammaglobulinemia. Specific tests for SLE include the following:
• *ANA, anti-deoxyribonucleic acid (DNA)*, and *lupus erythematosus cell tests* are positive in active SLE; because the anti-DNA test is rarely positive in other conditions, it's the most

specific test for SLE. However, if the patient is in remission, anti-DNA may be reduced or absent (it correlates with disease activity, especially renal involvement, and helps monitor the patient's response to therapy).

• *Urine studies* may show RBCs and WBCs, urine casts and sediment, and protein loss (more than 0.5 g/24 hours).

• *Blood studies* show decreased serum complement (C3 and C4) levels, which indicate active disease.

• *Chest X-ray* may show pleurisy or lupus pneumonitis.

• *Electrocardiogram* may show conduction defect with cardiac involvement or pericarditis.

• *Kidney biopsy* determines disease stage and extent of renal involvement.

Some patients show a positive *lupus anticoagulant test* and a positive *anticardiolipin test*. Such patients are prone to antiphospholipid syndrome (thrombosis, spontaneous abortion, and thrombocytopenia).

Treatment

Patients with mild disease require little or no medication. Nonsteroidal anti-inflammatory drugs, including aspirin, often control arthritis symptoms. Skin lesions need topical treatment. Corticosteroid creams, such as flurandrenolide, are recommended for acute lesions.

Refractory skin lesions are treated with intralesional corticosteroids or antimalarials, such as hydroxychloroquine and chloroquine. Because hydroxychloroquine and chloroquine can cause retinal damage, such treatment requires ophthalmologic examination every 6 months.

Corticosteroids remain the treatment of choice for systemic symptoms of SLE, for acute generalized exacerbations, or for serious disease related to vital organ systems, such as pleuritis, pericarditis, lupus nephritis, vasculitis, and CNS involvement. Initial doses equivalent to 60 mg or more of prednisone often bring noticeable improvement within 48 hours. As soon as symptoms are under control, steroid dosage is tapered. (Rising serum complement levels and decreasing anti-DNA titers indicate patient response.)

Diffuse proliferative glomerulonephritis, a major complication of SLE, requires treatment with large doses of steroids. If renal failure occurs, dialysis or kidney transplantation may be necessary. In some patients, cytotoxic drugs — such as azathioprine and cyclophosphamide — may delay or prevent deteriorating renal status. Antihypertensive drugs and dietary changes may also be warranted in renal disease.

The photosensitive patient should wear protective clothing (hat, sunglasses, long sleeves, slacks) and use a sunscreen containing para-aminobenzoic acid when exposed to the sun. Since SLE usually strikes women of childbearing age, questions associated with pregnancy often arise. The best evidence available indicates that a woman with SLE can have a safe, normal pregnancy if she has no serious renal or neurologic impairment.

Special considerations

• Watch for constitutional symptoms: joint pain or stiffness, weakness, fever, fatigue, and chills. Observe for dyspnea, chest pain, and any edema of the extremities. Note the size, type, and location of skin lesions. Check the patient's urine for hematuria, her scalp for hair loss, and her skin and mucous membranes for petechiae, bleeding, ulceration, pallor, and bruising.

• Provide a balanced diet. Foods high in protein, vitamins, and iron help maintain optimum nutrition and prevent anemia. However, renal involvement may mandate a low-sodium, low-protein diet.

• Urge the patient to get plenty of rest. Schedule diagnostic tests and procedures to allow adequate rest. Explain all tests and procedures. Tell the patient that several blood samples are needed initially, then periodically, to monitor progress.

• Apply heat packs to relieve joint pain and stiffness. Encourage regular exercise to maintain full range of motion (ROM) and prevent contractures. Teach ROM exercises, as well as body alignment and postural techniques. Arrange for physical therapy and occupational counseling as appropriate.

• Explain the expected benefits of prescribed medications, and watch for possible adverse reactions, especially when the patient is taking high doses of corticosteroids.

• For the patient receiving cyclophosphamide, encourage hydration and give mesna to prevent hemorrhagic cystitis and ondansetron to prevent nausea and vomiting.

• Monitor the patient's vital signs, intake and output, weight, and laboratory test results. Check pulse rates and observe for orthopnea. Check stools and GI secretions for blood.

• Observe for hypertension, weight gain, and other signs of renal involvement.

• Assess for signs of neurologic damage: personality change, paranoid or psychotic behavior, ptosis, or diplopia. Take seizure precautions. If Raynaud's phenomenon is present, warm and protect the patient's hands and feet.

• Offer cosmetic tips, such as suggesting the use of hypoallergenic makeup, and refer the patient to a hairdresser who specializes in scalp disorders.

• Advise the patient to purchase medications in quantity, if possible. Warn against "miracle" drugs for relief of arthritis symptoms.

• Refer the patient to her local chapter of the Lupus Foundation of America and the Arthritis Foundation as necessary.

Goodpasture's syndrome

In Goodpasture's syndrome, hemoptysis and rapidly progressive glomerulonephritis follow the deposition of antibodies against the alveolar and glomerular basement membranes. This syndrome may occur at any age but is most common in men between ages 20 and 30. The prognosis improves with aggressive immunosuppressive and antibiotic therapy and with dialysis or kidney transplantation.

Causes

Most cases of Goodpasture's syndrome have no precipitating events. The high incidence of the human leukocyte antigen (HLA) known as HLA-DRw2 in patients with Goodpasture's syndrome suggests a genetic predisposition. Abnormal production and deposition of antibodies against the glomerular basement membrane (GBM) and alveolar basement membrane activate the complement and inflammatory responses, resulting in glomerular and alveolar tissue damage.

Signs and symptoms

Goodpasture's syndrome may initially cause malaise, fatigue, and pallor associated with severe iron deficiency anemia. Pulmonary findings range from slight dyspnea and cough with blood-tinged sputum to hemoptysis and frank pulmonary hemorrhage. Subclinical pulmonary bleeding may precede overt hemorrhage and renal disease by months or years. Usually, renal findings are more subtle, although some patients note hematuria and peripheral edema.

Diagnosis

Confirmation of Goodpasture's syndrome requires measurement of circulating anti-GBM antibodies by radioimmunoassay and linear staining of the GBM and alveolar basement membrane by immunofluorescence.

Immunofluorescence of the alveolar basement membrane shows linear deposition of immunoglobulin, as well as the third component of complement and fibrinogen. Immunofluorescence of the GBM also shows linear deposition of immunoglobulin combined with circulating anti-GBM antibodies; this characteristic finding distinguishes Goodpasture's syndrome from other pulmonary-renal syndromes, such as Wegener's granulomatosis, polyarteritis, and systemic lupus erythematosus.

Lung biopsy shows interstitial and intra-alveolar hemorrhage with hemosiderin-laden macrophages. A chest X-ray reveals pulmonary infiltrates in a diffuse, nodular pattern, and a renal biopsy frequently shows focal necrotic lesions and cellular crescents.

Creatinine and blood urea nitrogen (BUN) levels typically increase two to three times above normal. Urinalysis may reveal red blood cells and cellular casts, which typify glomerular inflammation. Granular casts and proteinuria may also be observed.

Treatment

Effective treatment aims to remove antibodies by plasmapheresis and to suppress antibody production with immunosuppressive drugs. Patients with renal failure may benefit from dialysis or transplantation. Aggressive ultrafiltration helps relieve pulmonary edema that may aggravate pulmonary hemorrhage. High-dose I.V. steroids also help control pulmonary hemorrhage.

Special considerations

• Promote adequate oxygenation by elevating the head of the bed and administering humidified oxygen. Encourage the patient to conserve his energy. Assess respirations and breath sounds regularly; note sputum quantity and quality.

• Monitor the patient's vital signs, arterial blood gas levels, hematocrit, and coagulation studies.
• Transfuse blood and administer steroids as needed. Observe the patient closely for any adverse reactions associated with his medications.
• Assess renal function by monitoring symptomatology, intake and output, daily weight, creatinine clearance, and BUN and creatinine levels.
• Teach the patient and his family which signs and symptoms to expect and how to relieve them. Carefully describe other treatment measures such as dialysis.

Reiter's syndrome

A self-limiting syndrome associated with polyarthritis (its dominant feature), urethritis, balanitis, conjunctivitis, and mucocutaneous lesions, Reiter's syndrome appears to be related to infection, either venereal or enteric. This disease usually affects young men (ages 20 to 40); it's rarely seen in women and children.

Causes

Although the exact cause of Reiter's syndrome is unknown, most cases follow venereal or enteric infection. Because 75% to 85% of patients with Reiter's syndrome are positive for the HLA-B27 antigen, genetic susceptibility is likely. Reiter's syndrome has followed infections caused by *Mycoplasma, Shigella, Salmonella, Yersinia,* and *Chlamydia* organisms.

Signs and
symptoms

The patient with Reiter's syndrome may complain of dysuria, hematuria, urgent and frequent urination, and mucopurulent penile discharge, with swelling and reddening of the urethral meatus. Small painless ulcers may erupt on the glans penis (balanitis) and coalesce to form irregular patches that cover the penis and scrotum. The patient may also experience suprapubic pain, fever, and anorexia with weight loss. Reiter's syndrome may cause other genitourinary (GU) complications, such as prostatitis and hemorrhagic cystitis.

Arthritic symptoms usually follow GU or enteric symptoms and often last from 2 to 4 months. Asymmetrical and extremely variable polyarticular arthritis occurs most often and tends to develop in weight-bearing joints of the legs and sometimes in the sacroiliac joints of the lower back. The arthritis is usually acute, with warm, erythematous, and painful joints; but it may be mild, with minimal synovitis. Muscular atrophy is common near affected joints. Fingers and toes may swell and appear sausagelike.

Ocular symptoms include mild bilateral conjunctivitis, possibly complicated by keratitis, iritis, retinitis, or optic neuritis. In severe cases, burning, itching, and profuse mucopurulent discharge are possible.

In 30% of patients, skin lesions (keratoderma blennorrhagicum) develop 4 to 6 weeks after onset of other symptoms and may last for several weeks. These macular to hyperkeratotic lesions often resemble those of psoriasis. They occur most commonly on the palms and soles but can develop anywhere on the trunk, extremities, or scalp. Nails become thick, opaque, and brittle; keratic debris accumulates under the nails. In many patients, painless, transient ulcerations erupt on the buccal mucosa, palate, and tongue.

Diagnosis

Nearly all patients with Reiter's syndrome are positive for the HLA-B27 antigen and have an elevated white blood cell (WBC) count and erythrocyte sedimentation rate. Mild anemia may develop. Urethral discharge and synovial fluid contain many WBCs, mostly polymorphonuclear leukocytes; synovial fluid is high in complement and protein and is grossly purulent. Cultures of urethral discharge and synovial fluid rule out other causes such as gonococci.

During the first few weeks, X-rays are normal and may remain so, but some patients may show osteoporosis in inflamed areas. If inflammation persists, X-rays may show erosions of the small joints, periosteal proliferation (new bone formation) of involved joints, and calcaneal spurs.

Treatment

No specific treatment exists for Reiter's syndrome. Most patients recover in 2 to 16 weeks. About 50% of patients have recurring acute attacks, whereas the rest follow a chronic course, experiencing continued synovitis and sacroiliitis. In acute stages, limited weight-bearing or complete bed rest may be necessary.

Anti-inflammatory agents, the primary treatment, can be given to relieve discomfort and fever. Steroids may be used for persistent skin lesions; gold therapy and methotrexate or azathioprine, for bony erosion. Testing for human immuno-deficiency virus is needed before initiating steroid therapy. Physical therapy includes range-of-motion and strengthening exercises and the use of padded or supportive shoes to prevent contractures and foot deformities.

Special considerations

• Explain Reiter's syndrome to the patient. Discuss the medications and their possible adverse effects. Warn the patient to take medications with meals or milk to prevent GI bleeding.
• Encourage normal daily activity and moderate exercise. Suggest a firm mattress and encourage good posture and body mechanics.
• Arrange for occupational counseling if the patient has severe or chronic joint impairment.

Progressive systemic sclerosis

Also called CREST syndrome or scleroderma, progressive systemic sclerosis (PSS) is a diffuse connective tissue disease characterized by fibrotic, degenerative and, occasionally, inflammatory changes in skin, blood vessels, synovial membranes, skeletal muscles, and internal organs (especially the esophagus, GI tract, thyroid, heart, lungs, and kidneys). It affects women more frequently than men, especially between ages 30 and 50. Approximately 30% of patients with PSS die within 5 years of onset.

Causes

The cause of PSS is unknown. This disease occurs in distinctive forms:
• CREST syndrome is a benign form characterized by calcinosis, Raynaud's phenomenon, esophageal dysfunction, sclerodactyly, and telangiectasia.

• Diffuse systemic sclerosis is characterized by generalized skin thickening and invasion of internal organ systems.

• Localized scleroderma is characterized by patchy skin changes with a droplike appearance known as morphea.

• Linear scleroderma is characterized by a band of thickened skin on the face or extremities that severely damages underlying tissues, causing atrophy and deformity (most common in childhood).

Other forms include chemically induced localized scleroderma, eosinophilia-myalgia syndrome (recently associated with ingestion of L-tryptophan), toxic oil syndrome (associated with contaminated oil), and graft-versus-host disease.

Signs and symptoms

PSS typically begins with Raynaud's phenomenon — blanching, cyanosis, and erythema of the fingers and toes in response to stress or exposure to cold. Progressive phalangeal resorption may shorten the fingers.

Compromised circulation, which results from abnormal thickening of the arterial intima, may cause slowly healing ulcerations on the tips of the fingers or toes that may lead to gangrene. Raynaud's phenomenon may precede PSS by months or years.

Later symptoms include pain, stiffness, and swelling of the fingers and joints. Skin thickening produces taut, shiny skin over the entire hand and forearm. Facial skin also becomes tight and inelastic, causing a masklike appearance and "pinching" of the mouth. As tightening progresses, contractures may develop.

GI dysfunction causes frequent reflux, heartburn, dysphagia, and bloating after meals. These symptoms may cause the patient to decrease food intake and lose weight. Other GI effects include abdominal distention, diarrhea, constipation, and malodorous, floating stools.

In advanced disease, cardiac and pulmonary fibrosis produce dysrhythmias and dyspnea. Renal involvement is usually accompanied by malignant hypertension, the cause of death.

Diagnosis

Typical cutaneous changes provide the first clue to diagnosis. Results of diagnostic tests include the following:

• *Blood studies* show slightly elevated erythrocyte sedimentation rate, positive rheumatoid factor in 25% to 35% of patients, and positive antinuclear antibody test.

• *Urinalysis* shows proteinuria, microscopic hematuria, and casts (with renal involvement).

• *Hand X-rays* show terminal phalangeal tuft resorption, subcutaneous calcification, and joint space narrowing and erosion

• *Chest X-rays* show bilateral basilar pulmonary fibrosis.

• *GI X-rays* show distal esophageal hypomotility and stricture, duodenal loop dilation, small-bowel malabsorption pattern, and large diverticula.

• *Pulmonary function studies* show decreased diffusion and vital capacity.

• *Electrocardiogram* shows possible nonspecific abnormalities related to myocardial fibrosis.

• *Skin biopsy* may show changes consistent with the progress of the disease, such as marked thickening of the dermis and occlusive vessel changes.

Treatment

Currently, no cure exists for PSS. Treatment aims to preserve normal body functions and minimize complications. Use of immunosuppressives, such as chlorambucil, is a common palliative measure. (FK-506 is experimental.) Corticosteroids and colchicine have been used experimentally and seem to stabilize symptoms; D-penicillamine may be helpful. Blood platelet levels need to be monitored throughout drug therapy. Other treatments vary according to the following symptoms:

• *Raynaud's phenomenon:* various vasodilators and antihypertensive agents (such as methyldopa or calcium channel blockers), intermittent cervical sympathetic blockade or, rarely, thoracic sympathectomy.

• *chronic digital ulcerations:* a digital plaster cast to immobilize the affected area, minimize trauma, and maintain cleanliness; possibly surgical debridement.

• *esophagitis with stricture:* antacids; cimetidine; a soft, bland diet; and periodic esophageal dilation.

• *small-bowel involvement* (diarrhea, pain, malabsorption, weight loss): broad-spectrum antibiotics, such as erythromycin or tetracycline, to counteract bacterial overgrowth in the duodenum and jejunum related to hypomotility.

• *scleroderma kidney* (with malignant hypertension and impending renal failure): dialysis, antihypertensives, and calcium channel blockers.
• *hand debilitation:* physical therapy to maintain function and promote muscle strength, heat therapy to relieve joint stiffness, and patient teaching to make performance of daily activities easier.

Special considerations

• Assess motion restrictions, pain, vital signs, intake and output, respiratory function, and daily weight.
• Because of compromised circulation, warn against fingerstick blood tests.
• Remember that air conditioning may aggravate Raynaud's phenomenon.
• Help the patient and her family adjust to the patient's new body image and to the limitations and dependency these changes cause.
• Teach the patient to avoid fatigue by pacing activities and organizing schedules to include necessary rest.
• The patient and her family need to accept the fact that this condition is incurable. Encourage them to express their feelings, and help them cope with their fears and frustrations by offering information about the disease, its treatment, and relevant diagnostic tests.
• Whenever possible, let the patient participate in treatment by measuring her intake and output, planning her own diet, assisting in dialysis, giving herself heat therapy, and doing the prescribed exercises.

Polymyositis and dermatomyositis

Diffuse, inflammatory myopathies of unknown cause, polymyositis and dermatomyositis produce symmetrical weakness of striated muscle – primarily proximal muscles of the shoulder and pelvic girdle, neck, and pharynx. In dermatomyositis, such muscle weakness is accompanied by cutaneous involvement. These diseases usually progress slowly, with frequent exacerbations and remissions. They occur twice as often in women as in men (with the exception of dermatomyositis associated with cancer, which is most common in men over age 40).

Generally, prognosis worsens with age. The 7-year survival rate for adults is approximately 60%, with death often occurring from associated cancer, respiratory disease, heart failure, or adverse effects of therapy (corticosteroids and immunosuppressives). Up to 90% of affected children regain normal function if properly treated; if untreated, childhood dermatomyositis may progress rapidly to disabling contractures and muscular atrophy.

Causes

Although the cause of polymyositis remains puzzling, researchers believe that it may result from an autoimmune reaction. Presumably, the patient's T cells inappropriately recognize muscle fiber antigens as foreign and attack muscle tissue, causing diffuse or focal muscle fiber degeneration. (Regeneration of new muscle cells then follows, producing remission.) Polymyositis and dermatomyositis may be associated with other disorders such as allergic reactions; systemic lupus erythematosus (SLE); scleroderma; rheumatoid arthritis; Sjögren's syndrome; carcinomas of the lung, breast, or other organs; D-penicillamine administration; or systemic viral infection.

Signs and symptoms

Polymyositis begins acutely or insidiously with muscle weakness, tenderness, and discomfort. It affects proximal muscles (shoulder, pelvic girdle) more often than distal muscles. Muscle weakness impairs performance of ordinary activities. The patient may have trouble getting up from a chair, combing her hair, reaching into a high cupboard, climbing stairs, or even raising her head from a pillow. Other muscular symptoms that the patient may have include an inability to move against resistance, proximal dysphagia, and dysphonia.

In dermatomyositis, an erythematous rash usually erupts on the face, neck, upper back, chest, and arms and around the nail beds. A characteristic heliotropic rash appears on the eyelids, accompanied by periorbital edema. Grotton's papules (violet, flat-topped lesions) may appear on the interphalangeal joints.

Diagnosis

Muscle biopsy shows necrosis, degeneration, regeneration, and interstitial chronic lymphocytic infiltration. Appropriate laboratory tests differentiate polymyositis from diseases that cause similar muscular or cutaneous symptoms, such as muscular dystrophy, advanced trichinosis, psoriasis, seborrheic dermatitis, and SLE.

Typical laboratory test results in polymyositis include an elevated erythrocyte sedimentation rate; elevated white blood cell count; elevated muscle enzyme levels (creatine kinase, aldolase, aspartate aminotransferase) not attributable to hemolysis of red blood cells or hepatic or other diseases; an increased urine creatine level (more than 150 mg/24 hours); a decreased creatinine level; electromyography showing polyphasic short-duration potentials, fibrillation (positive spike waves), and bizarre high-frequency repetitive changes; and positive antinuclear antibodies.

Treatment

High-dose corticosteroid therapy relieves inflammation and lowers muscle enzyme levels. Within 2 to 6 weeks following treatment, serum muscle enzyme levels usually return to normal and muscle strength improves, permitting a gradual tapering of corticosteroid dosage. If the patient responds poorly to corticosteroids, treatment may include cytotoxic or immunosuppressive drugs, such as cyclophosphamide, given by intermittent I.V. or orally, once a day.

Supportive therapy includes bed rest during the acute phase, range-of-motion (ROM) exercises to prevent contractures, analgesics and application of heat to relieve painful muscle spasms, and diphenhydramine to relieve itching. Patients over age 40 need a thorough assessment for coexisting cancers.

Special considerations

• Assess the patient's level of pain, muscle weakness, and range of motion daily. Administer analgesics as needed.
• If the patient is confined to bed, prevent pressure ulcers by giving good skin care. To prevent footdrop and contractures, apply high-topped sneakers, and assist with passive ROM-exercises at least four times daily. Teach the patient's family how to perform these exercises on the patient.
• If 24-hour urine collection is necessary for monitoring creatine or creatinine levels, make sure that your coworkers understand the procedure. When you assist with muscle bi-

opsy, make sure that the biopsy is not taken from an area of recent needle insertion, such as an injection or electromyography site.

• If the patient has a skin rash, warn her against scratching, which may cause infection. If antipruritic medication doesn't relieve severe itching, apply tepid sponges or compresses.

• Encourage the patient to feed and dress herself to the best of her ability but to ask for help when needed. Advise her to pace her activities to counteract muscle weakness. Encourage her to express her anxiety. Ease the patient's fear of dependence by reassuring her that muscle weakness is probably temporary.

• Explain the disease to the patient and her family. Prepare them for diagnostic procedures and possible adverse effects of corticosteroid therapy (weight gain, hirsutism, hypertension, edema, amenorrhea, purplish striae, glycosuria, acne, easy bruising). Advise a low-sodium diet to prevent fluid retention. Emphatically warn against abruptly discontinuing corticosteroids. Reassure the patient that steroid-induced weight gain will diminish when the drug is discontinued.

Vasculitis

This disorder includes a broad spectrum of disorders characterized by inflammation and necrosis of the blood vessels. The clinical effects of vasculitis depend on the vessels involved and reflect tissue ischemia caused by blood flow obstruction. The prognosis is also variable. For example, hypersensitivity vasculitis is usually a benign disorder limited to the skin, but more extensive polyarteritis nodosa can be rapidly fatal.

Vasculitis can occur at any age, except for mucocutaneous lymph node syndrome, which occurs only during childhood. Vasculitis may be a primary disorder or secondary to other disorders such as rheumatoid arthritis or systemic lupus erythematosus.

Causes

Exactly how vascular damage develops in vasculitis isn't well understood. Current theory holds that it's initiated by an excessive level of antigen in the circulation, which triggers the formation of soluble antigen-antibody complexes. These complexes cannot be effectively cleared by the reticuloendothelial system and so are deposited in blood vessel walls (Type III hypersensitivity). Increased vascular permeability associated with release of vasoactive amines by platelets and basophils enhances such deposition. The deposited complexes activate the complement cascade, resulting in chemotaxis of neutrophils, which release lysosomal enzymes. In turn, these enzymes cause vessel damage and necrosis, which may precipitate thrombosis, occlusion, hemorrhage, and tissue ischemia.

Another mechanism that may contribute to vascular damage is the cell-mediated (T-cell) immune response. In this response, circulating antigen triggers the release of soluble mediators by sensitized lymphocytes, which attract macrophages. The macrophages release intracellular enzymes, which cause vascular damage. They can also transform into the epithelioid and multinucleated giant cells that typify the granulomatous vasculitides. Phagocytosis of immune complexes by macrophages enhances granuloma formation.

Signs, symptoms, and diagnosis

Clinical effects of vasculitis and laboratory procedures used to confirm the diagnosis depend on the blood vessels involved. See *Distinguishing among types of vasculitis*, pages 102 and 103, for signs, symptoms, and diagnostic criteria specific to each type of vasculitis.

Treatment

In vasculitis, treatment aims to minimize irreversible tissue damage associated with ischemia. In primary vasculitis, treatment may involve removal of an offending antigen or use of anti-inflammatory or immunosuppressive drugs. For example, antigenic drugs, food, and other environmental substances should be identified and eliminated, if possible. Drug therapy in primary vasculitis frequently involves low-dose cyclophosphamide (2 mg/kg P.O. daily) with daily corticosteroids. In rapidly fulminant vasculitis, cyclophosphamide dosage may be increased to 4 mg/kg daily for the first 2 to 3 days, followed by the regular dose. Prednisone should be

(Text continues on page 104.)

Distinguishing among types of vasculitis

TYPE	VESSELS INVOLVED
Polyarteritis nodosa	Small- to medium-sized arteries throughout body. Lesions tend to be segmental, occur at bifurcations and branchings of arteries, and spread distally to arterioles. In severe cases, lesions circumferentially involve adjacent veins.
Allergic angiitis and granulomatosis (Churg-Strauss syndrome)	Small- to medium-sized arteries and small vessels (arterioles, capillaries, and venules), mainly of the lungs but also of other organs
Polyangiitis overlap syndrome	Small- to medium-sized arteries and small vessels (arterioles, capillaries, venules) of the lungs and of other organs
Wegener's granulomatosis	Small- to medium-sized vessels of the respiratory tract and kidneys
Temporal arteritis	Medium- to large-sized arteries, most commonly branches of the carotid artery
Takayasu's arteritis (aortic arch syndrome)	Medium- to large-sized arteries, particularly the aortic arch and its branches and, possibly, the pulmonary artery
Hypersensitivity vasculitis	Small vessels, especially of the skin
Mucocutaneous lymph node syndrome (Kawasaki disease)	Small- to medium-sized vessels, primarily of the lymph nodes; may progress to involve coronary arteries
Behçet's syndrome	Small vessels, primarily of the mouth and genitalia but also of the eyes, skin, joints, GI tract, and central nervous system

SIGNS AND SYMPTOMS	DIAGNOSIS
Hypertension, abdominal pain, myalgias, headache, joint pain, weakness	History of symptoms. Elevated erythrocyte sedimentation rate (ESR), leukocytosis, anemia, thrombocytosis, depressed C3 complement, rheumatoid factor > 1:60, circulating immune complexes. Tissue biopsy shows necrotizing vasculitis.
Resembles polyarteritis nodosa with hallmark of severe pulmonary involvement	History of asthma. Eosinophilia; tissue biopsy shows granulomatous inflammation with eosinophilic infiltration.
Combines symptoms of polyarteritis nodosa and allergic angiitis and granulomatosis	Possible history of allergy. Eosinophilia; tissue biopsy shows granulomatous inflammation with eosinophilic infiltration.
Fever, pulmonary congestion, cough, malaise, anorexia, weight loss, mild to severe hematuria	Tissue biopsy shows necrotizing vasculitis with granulomatous inflammation. Leukocytosis; elevated ESR, IgA, and IgG; low titer rheumatoid factor; circulating immune complexes; antineutrophil cytoplasmic antibody in more than 90% of patients
Fever, myalgia, jaw claudication, visual changes, headache (associated with polymyalgia rheumatica syndrome)	Decreased hemoglobin; elevated ESR; tissue biopsy shows panarteritis with infiltration of mononuclear cells, giant cells within vessel wall, fragmentation of internal elastic lamina, and proliferation of intima.
Malaise, pallor, nausea, night sweats, arthralgias, anorexia, weight loss, pain or paresthesia distal to affected area, bruits, loss of distal pulses, syncope and, if carotid artery is involved, diplopia and transient blindness. May progress to congestive heart failure or cerebrovascular accident.	Decreased hemoglobin; leukocytosis; positive lupus erythematosus cell preparation and elevated ESR. Arteriography shows calcification and obstruction of affected vessels. Tissue biopsy shows inflammation of adventitia and intima of vessels, and thickening of vessel walls.
Palpable purpura, papules, nodules, vesicles, bullae, ulcers, or chronic or recurrent urticaria	History of exposure to antigen, such as a microorganism or drug. Tissue biopsy shows leukocytoclastic angiitis, usually in postcapillary venules, with infiltration of polymorphonuclear leukocytes, fibrinoid necrosis, and extravasation of erthyrocytes.
Fever; nonsuppurative cervical adenitis; edema; congested conjunctivae; erythema of oral cavity, lips, and palms; and desquamation of fingertips. May progress to arthritis, myocarditis, pericarditis, myocardial infarction, and cardiomegaly.	History of symptoms. Elevated ESR; tissue biopsy shows intimal proliferation and infiltration of vessel walls with mononuclear cells. Echocardiography necessary.
Recurrent oral ulcers, eye lesions, genital lesions, and cutaneous lesions	History of symptoms.

given in a dose of 1 mg/kg daily in divided doses for 7 to 10 days, with consolidation to a single morning dose by 2 to 3 weeks. When the vasculitis appears to be in remission or when prescribed cytotoxic drugs take full effect, corticosteroids are tapered to a single daily dose and then to an alternate-day schedule that may continue for 3 to 6 months before steroids are slowly discontinued.

In secondary vasculitis, treatment focuses on the underlying disorder.

Special considerations

- Assess for dry nasal mucosa in patients with Wegener's granulomatosis. Instill nose drops to lubricate the mucosa and help diminish crusting. Or irrigate the nasal passages with warm 0.9% sodium chloride solution.
- Monitor vital signs. Use a Doppler ultrasonic flowmeter, if available, to auscultate blood pressure in patients with Takayasu's arteritis, whose peripheral pulses are frequently difficult to palpate.
- Monitor the patient's intake and output. Check daily for edema. Keep the patient well-hydrated (3 liters daily) to reduce the risk of hemorrhagic cystitis associated with cyclophosphamide therapy.
- Provide emotional support to help the patient and his family cope with an altered body image—the result of the disorder or its therapy. (For example, Wegener's granulomatosis may be associated with saddle nose; steroids may cause weight gain; and cyclophosphamide may cause alopecia.)
- Teach the patient how to recognize adverse effects of these medications. Monitor the patient's white blood cell count during cyclophosphamide therapy to prevent severe leukopenia.

Self-test questions

You can quickly review your comprehension of autoimmune disorders by answering the following questions. The correct answers to these questions and their rationales appear on pages 154 to 156.

Case history
questions

Jane Addis, a 34-year-old librarian, is suspected of having rheumatoid arthritis (RA) based on her demonstrating typical signs and symptoms for the past 2 months.

1. Ms. Addis initially experienced:
   a. nonspecific symptoms.
   b. generalized morning stiffness.
   c. tender, painful joints.
   d. swollen, congested joints.

2. Joints affected by RA, besides those of the hands, include the:
   a. hips and knees.
   b. wrists, elbows, knees, and ankles.
   c. shoulders, hips, knees, and ankles.
   d. costovertebral and sternomanubrial joints.

3. Joint deformities in RA include:
   a. Heberden's nodes.
   b. ulnar drift.
   c. Bouchard's nodes.
   d. rheumatoid nodules.

4. The mainstay of RA therapy is:
   a. nonsteroidal anti-inflammatory drugs, such as indomethacin and ibuprofen.
   b. immunosuppressives, such as methotrexate and azathioprine.
   c. corticosteroids, such as prednisone.
   d. salicylates.

5. Which of these drug classes is contraindicated in psoriatic arthritis?
   a. NSAIDs
   b. Gold salts
   c. Systemic corticosteroids
   d. Antimalarials

6. Which of the following drug classes is also useful in managing ankylosing spondylitis?

    a. Anti-inflammatory analgesics, such as aspirin and indomethacin
    b. Immunosuppressives, such as methotrexate
    c. Corticosteroids, such as prednisone
    d. Antimalarials, such as hydroxychloroquine

7. Sjögren's syndrome is an autoimmune rheumatic disorder characterized by:
    a. urethritis, arthritis, and conjunctivitis.
    b. nail changes, including pitting, transverse ridging, and keratosis.
    c. iridocyclitis.
    d. diminished lacrimal and salivary gland secretion.

Tina Rogers was diagnosed with systemic lupus erythematosus as a teenager, following a severe streptococcal throat infection treated with penicillin.

8. Tina's symptoms included fever, weight loss, malaise, and fatigue; however, she did not develop the classic:
    a. polyarthralgia.
    b. butterfly rash over the nose and cheeks.
    c. vasculitis.
    d. Raynaud's phenomenon.

9. In addition to demonstrating a positive anti-deoxyribonucleic acid test, Tina's tests indicated renal involvement. Urine studies showed:
    a. large numbers of red blood cells.
    b. elevated porphyrin levels.
    c. cellular casts and profuse proteinuria.
    d. decreased creatinine levels.

10. In an attempt to delay renal deterioration, Tina was prescribed:
    a. large doses of prednisone.
    b. fosinopril.
    c. a low-protein, high-caloric diet.
    d. azathioprine.

CHAPTER 4

Immunodeficiency

Caused by an absent or a depressed immune response and manifested in various forms, immunodeficiency disorders include X-linked infantile hypogammaglobulinemia, common variable immunodeficiency, selective immunoglobulin A deficiency, DiGeorge's syndrome, acquired immunodeficiency syndrome, chronic mucocutaneous candidiasis, chronic fatigue and immune dysfunction syndrome, immunodeficiency with eczema and thrombocytopenia, ataxia-telangiectasia, chronic granulomatous disease, Chédiak-Higashi syndrome, severe combined immunodeficiency disease, and complement deficiencies.

X-linked infantile hypogammaglobulinemia

Also known as Bruton's agammaglobulinemia, X-linked infantile hypogammaglobulinemia is a congenital disorder in which all five classes of immunoglobulin—immunoglobulin M (IgM), IgG, IgA, IgD, and IgE—and circulating B cells are absent or deficient but T cells are intact. Affecting males almost exclusively, this disorder occurs in 1 in 50,000 to 100,000 births and causes severe, recurrent infections during infancy. Prognosis is good with early treatment, except in infants who develop polio or persistent viral infection. Infection usually causes some permanent damage, especially in the neurologic or respiratory system.

Causes

In this disease, B cells and B-cell precursors may be present in the bone marrow and peripheral blood, but a mutation in the B-cell protein tyrosine kinase causes failure of B cells to mature and secrete immunoglobulin.

Normal levels of immunoglobulins

AGE	mg/dl	% OF ADULT LEVEL
Newborn	6 to 16	6 to 16
1 to 3 mo	19 to 41	19 to 41
4 to 6 mo	26 to 60	26 to 60
7 to 12 mo	31 to 77	32 to 78
13 to 24 mo	35 to 81	36 to 82
25 to 36 mo	42 to 80	43 to 81
3 to 5 yr	38 to 74	39 to 75
6 to 8 yr	40 to 90	41 to 91
9 to 11 yr	46 to 112	47 to 100
12 to 16 yr	39 to 79	40 to 80
Adults	72 to 126	

Signs and symptoms

Typically, the infant with X-linked hypogammaglobulinemia is asymptomatic until age 6 months, when transplacental maternal immunoglobulins, which to that point have provided immune response, have been depleted. Then he develops recurrent bacterial otitis media, pneumonia, dermatitis, bronchitis, and meningitis – usually caused by pneumococci, streptococci, or *Haemophilus influenzae* or other gram-negative organisms. Purulent conjunctivitis, abnormal dental caries, and polyarthritis resembling rheumatoid arthritis may also occur. Severe malabsorption associated with infestation by *Giardia lamblia* may result in retarded development. Despite recurrent infections, lymphadenopathy and splenomegaly are usually absent.

Diagnosis

Diagnosis of X-linked hypogammaglobulinemia may be especially difficult, because recurrent infections are common even in normal infants (many of whom don't start producing their own antibodies until age 18 to 20 months). It rests on the detection of absent or decreased IgM, IgA, and IgG in the serum by immunoelectrophoresis. (See *Normal levels of immunoglobulins*.) However, diagnosis by this method usually isn't possible until the infant is 9 months old. Antigenic stimulation confirms an inability to produce specific antibodies, although cellular immunity remains intact.

Treatment

Treatment aims to prevent or control infections and to boost the patient's immune response. Injection of immune globulin helps maintain immune response. Because immune globulin is composed primarily of IgG, the patient may also need fresh frozen plasma infusions to provide IgA and IgM. Unfortunately, mucosal secretory IgA cannot be replaced by therapy, resulting in frequent crippling pulmonary disease. Judicious use of antibiotics also helps combat infection; in some cases, chronic broad-spectrum antibiotics may be indicated.

Special considerations

• Because immune globulin injections are painful, give them deep into a large muscle mass, such as the gluteal or thigh muscles, and massage well.
• If the dosage is more than 1.5 ml, divide it and inject it into more than one site; for frequent injections, rotate the injection sites.
• To help prevent severe infection, teach the patient and his family how to recognize its early signs and to report them promptly.
• Advise the patient and his family to have cuts and scrapes cleaned immediately. Warn them to avoid crowds and persons who have active infections.
• During acute infection, monitor the patient closely.
• Maintain adequate nutrition and hydration, and perform chest physiotherapy if required.
• As always, carefully explain all treatment measures and make sure the patient and his family understand the disorder.
• Suggest genetic counseling if parents have questions about vulnerability of their future offspring.

Common variable immunodeficiency

Also called acquired hypogammaglobulinemia and agammaglobulinemia with immunoglobulin-bearing B cells, common variable immunodeficiency is characterized by progressive deterioration of B-cell (humoral) immunity, resulting in increased susceptibility to infection. Unlike X-linked hypogammaglobulinemia, this disorder usually causes symptoms after infancy and childhood, between ages 25 and 40. It affects males and females equally and usually doesn't interfere with normal life span or with normal pregnancy and offspring.

Causes

What causes common variable immunodeficiency is unknown. Most patients have a normal circulating B-cell count but defective synthesis or release of immunoglobulins. Many also exhibit progressive deterioration of T-cell (cell-mediated) immunity revealed by delayed hypersensitivity skin testing.

Signs and symptoms

In common variable immunodeficiency, pyogenic bacterial infections are characteristic, but tend to be chronic rather than acute (as in X-linked hypogammaglobulinemia). Recurrent sinopulmonary infections, chronic bacterial conjunctivitis, and malabsorption (often associated with infestation by *Giardia lamblia*) are usually the first clues to immunodeficiency.

Common variable immunodeficiency may be associated with autoimmune diseases, such as systemic lupus erythematosus, rheumatoid arthritis, hemolytic anemia, and pernicious anemia, and with cancer, such as leukemia and lymphoma.

Diagnosis

Characteristic diagnostic markers in this disorder are decreased serum immunoglobulin M (IgM), A (IgA), and G (IgG) detected by immunoelectrophoresis, along with a normal circulating B-cell count. Antigenic stimulation confirms an inability to produce specific antibodies; cell-mediated immunity may be intact or delayed. X-rays usually show signs of chronic lung disease or sinusitis.

Treatment

Treatment and care for patients with common variable immunodeficiency are essentially the same as for X-linked hypogammaglobulinemia.

Injection of immune globulin (usually weekly to monthly) helps maintain immune response. Antibiotics are the mainstay for combating infection. Regular X-rays and pulmonary function studies help monitor infection in the lungs; chest physiotherapy may be ordered to forestall or help clear such infection.

Special
considerations

• Because immune globulin injections are painful, give them deep into a large muscle mass, such as the gluteal or thigh muscles, and massage well.
• If the dosage is more than 1.5 ml, divide the dose and inject it into more than one site; for frequent injections, rotate the injection sites.
• Because immune globulin is composed primarily of IgG, the patient may also need fresh frozen plasma infusions to provide IgA and IgM.
• To help prevent severe infection, teach the patient and his family how to recognize its early signs.
• Warn the patient and his family to avoid crowds and persons who have active infections.
• Stress the importance of good nutrition and regular follow-up care.

Selective IgA deficiency

Selective immunoglobulin A (IgA) deficiency, which is also called Janeway Type 3 dysgammaglobulinemia, is the most common immunoglobulin deficiency. It affects as many as 1 in 800 persons. IgA — the major immunoglobulin in human saliva, nasal and bronchial fluids, and intestinal secretions — guards against bacterial and viral reinfections. Consequently, IgA deficiency leads to chronic sinopulmonary infections, GI diseases, and other disorders. The prognosis is good for patients who receive the appropriate treatment, especially if they are free of associated disorders. Such patients have been known to survive to age 70.

Causes

IgA deficiency seems to be linked to autosomal dominant or recessive inheritance. The presence of normal numbers of peripheral blood lymphocytes carrying IgA receptors and of normal amounts of other immunoglobulins suggests that B cells may not be secreting IgA. In an occasional patient, suppressor T cells appear to inhibit IgA. IgA deficiency also seems related to autoimmune disorders, because many patients with rheumatoid arthritis or systemic lupus erythematosus are also IgA deficient. Some drugs, such as anticonvulsants, may cause transient IgA deficiency.

Signs and symptoms

Some IgA-deficient patients have no symptoms, possibly because they have extra amounts of low-molecular-weight IgM, which takes over IgA's function and helps maintain immune defenses. Among patients who do develop symptoms, chronic sinopulmonary infection is most common. Other effects are respiratory allergy, often triggered by infection; GI tract diseases, such as celiac disease, ulcerative colitis, and regional enteritis; autoimmune diseases, such as rheumatoid arthritis, systemic lupus erythematosus, immune anemia, and chronic hepatitis; and malignant tumors, such as squamous cell carcinoma of the lungs, reticulum cell sarcoma, and thymoma. Age of onset varies. Some IgA-deficient children with recurrent respiratory disease and middle-ear inflammation may begin to synthesize IgA spontaneously as recurrent infections subside and their condition improves.

Diagnosis

Immunologic analysis of IgA-deficient patients shows serum IgA levels below 5 mg/dl. While IgA is usually absent from secretions in IgA-deficient patients, levels may be normal in rare cases. IgE is normal, while IgM may be normal or elevated in serum and secretions. Normally absent low-molecular-weight IgM may be present.

Tests may also indicate autoantibodies and antibodies against IgG (rheumatoid factor), IgM, and bovine milk. Cell-mediated immunity is usually normal, and most circulating B cells appear normal.

Treatment

Selective IgA deficiency has no known cure. Treatment aims to control symptoms of associated diseases, such as respiratory and GI infections, and is generally the same as for a patient with normal IgA, with one exception: *Don't* give an IgA-deficient patient immune globulin, because sensitization may lead to anaphylaxis during future administration of blood products.

Special considerations

• If transfusion with blood products is necessary, minimize the risk of adverse reaction by using washed red blood cells, or avoid the reaction completely by crossmatching the patient's blood with that of an IgA-deficient donor.
• Because this is a lifelong disorder, teach the patient to prevent infection, to recognize its early signs, and to seek treatment promptly.

DiGeorge's syndrome

DiGeorge's syndrome (congenital thymic hypoplasia or aplasia) is a disorder known typically by the partial or total absence of cell-mediated immunity that results from a deficiency of T lymphocytes. It characteristically produces life-threatening hypocalcemia that may be associated with cardiovascular and facial anomalies. Patients rarely live beyond age 2 without fetal thymic transplant; however, prognosis improves when fetal thymic transplant, correction of hypocalcemia, and repair of cardiac anomalies are possible.

Causes

DiGeorge's syndrome is probably caused by abnormal fetal development of the third and fourth pharyngeal pouches (12th week of gestation) that interferes with the formation of the thymus. As a result, the thymus is completely or partially absent and abnormally located, causing deficient cell-mediated immunity. (See *Role of the thymus in immune response,* page 114.) This syndrome has been associated with maternal alcoholism and resultant fetal alcohol syndrome.

Role of the thymus in immune response

The thymus provides an environment in which T cells develop and learn to distinguish self from nonself during fetal and early postnatal stages. Most cells that enter the thymus are destroyed. T-cell clones that react strongly to self and those that do not recognize self are deleted (negative selection). T-cell clones that recognize self but don't react strongly against self are positively selected.

After early life, mature T cells reside primarily in peripheral lymph organs and recirculate in blood and lymph.

Signs and symptoms

Symptoms are usually obvious at birth or shortly thereafter. An infant with DiGeorge's syndrome may have low-set ears, notched ear pinnae, a fish-shaped mouth, an undersized jaw, and abnormally wide-set eyes (hypertelorism) with anti-mongoloid eyelid formation (downward slant). Cardiovascular abnormalities include great blood vessel anomalies (these may also develop soon after birth) and tetralogy of Fallot. The thymus may be absent or underdeveloped and abnormally located. An infant with thymic hypoplasia (rather than aplasia) may experience a spontaneous return of cell-mediated immunity but can develop severe T-cell deficiencies later in life, allowing exaggerated susceptibility to viral, fungal, or bacterial infections, which may be overwhelming. Typically, hypoparathyroidism, usually associated with Di-George's syndrome, causes tetany, hyperphosphoremia, and hypocalcemia. Hypocalcemia develops early and is both life-threatening and unusually resistant to treatment. It can lead to seizures, central nervous system damage, and early congestive heart failure.

Diagnosis

Immediate diagnosis is difficult unless the infant shows typical facial anomalies—normally the first clues to the disorder. Definitive diagnosis depends on successful treatment of hypocalcemia and other life-threatening birth defects during the first few weeks of life. Such diagnosis rests on proof of decreased or absent T lymphocytes (sheep cell test, lymphopenia) and of an absent thymus (chest X-ray). Immunoglobulin assays are useless, because antibodies present are usually from maternal circulation.

Additional tests showing low serum calcium, elevated serum phosphorus, and missing parathyroid hormone confirm hypoparathyroidism.

Treatment

Life-threatening hypocalcemia must be treated immediately, but it's unusually resistant and requires aggressive treatment—for example, with a rapid I.V. infusion of 10% solution of calcium gluconate. After hypocalcemia is under control, fetal thymic transplant may restore normal cell-mediated immunity. Cardiac anomalies require surgical repair when possible.

Special considerations

• During I.V. infusion with 10% solution of calcium gluconate, monitor heart rate and watch to avoid infiltration.
• Remember that calcium supplements *must* be given with vitamin D, or sometimes also with parathyroid hormone, to ensure effective calcium utilization.
• A patient with DiGeorge's syndrome also needs a low-phosphorus diet and preventive measures for infection.
• Teach the mother of such an infant to watch for signs of infection and, when needed, seek treatment immediately; to keep the infant away from crowds or any other potential sources of infection; and to provide good hygiene and adequate nutrition and hydration.

Acquired immunodeficiency syndrome

Although acquired immunodeficiency syndrome (AIDS) is characterized by progressive destruction of cell-mediated (T-cell) immunity, it also affects humoral immunity and even autoimmunity because of the central role of the CD4+ T lymphocyte in immune reactions. The resultant immunodeficiency makes the patient susceptible to opportunistic infections, unusual cancers, and other abnormalities that define AIDS. This syndrome was first described by the Centers for Disease Control and Prevention (CDC) in 1981. Since then, the CDC has declared a case surveillance definition for AIDS and modified it several times, most recently in 1993.

A retrovirus, the human immunodeficiency virus (HIV) Type I is the primary etiologic factor agent. Transmission of HIV occurs by contact with infected blood or body fluids. Because of similar routes of transmission, AIDS shares epidemiologic patterns with hepatitis B and sexually transmitted diseases.

The natural history of AIDS infection begins with infection by the HIV retrovirus, which is detectable only by laboratory tests, and ends with the severely immunocompromised, terminal stage of this disease. Depending on individual variations and the presence of cofactors that influence progression, the time elapsed from acute HIV infection to the appearance of symptoms, to diagnosis of AIDS, and eventually to death varies greatly. Current antiretroviral therapy (for example, with zidovudine) and treatment and prophylaxis of common opportunistic infections can delay the progression of HIV disease and prolong survival.

Causes

AIDS results from infection with HIV, which strikes cells bearing the CD4 antigen. This antigen (normally a receptor for major histocompatibility complex molecules) serves as a receptor for the retrovirus and lets it enter the cell. HIV prefers to infect the $CD4^+$ lymphocyte but may also infect other $CD4^+$ antigen-bearing cells of the GI tract, uterocervical cells, and neuroglial cells. After invading a cell, HIV replicates, leading to cell death, or becomes latent. HIV infection leads to profound pathology, either directly, through destruction of $CD4^+$ cells, other immune cells, and neuroglial cells, or indirectly, through the secondary effects of $CD4^+$ T-cell dysfunction and resultant immunosuppression. The infection process takes three forms: immunodeficiency (opportunistic infections and unusual cancers), autoimmunity (lymphoid interstitial pneumonitis, arthritis, hypergammaglobulinemia, and production of autoimmune antibodies), and neurologic dysfunction (AIDS dementia complex, HIV encephalopathy, and peripheral neuropathies).

HIV is transmitted by direct inoculation during intimate sexual contact, especially associated with the mucosal trauma of receptive rectal intercourse; transfusion of contaminated blood or blood products; sharing of contaminated needles; or transplacental or postpartum transmission from infected mother to fetus (by cervical or blood contact at delivery and in breast milk). Accumulating evidence suggests that HIV is not transmitted by casual household or social contact. The average time between exposure to the virus and diagnosis of AIDS is 8 to 10 years, but shorter and longer incubation times have also been recorded.

Signs and symptoms

After a high-risk exposure and inoculation, the infected person usually experiences a mononucleosis-like syndrome, which may be attributed to a flu or other virus and then may remain asymptomatic for years. In this latent stage, the only sign of HIV infection is laboratory evidence of seroconversion. When symptoms appear, they may take many forms: persistent generalized adenopathy, nonspecific symptoms (weight loss, fatigue, night sweats, fevers), neurologic symptoms resulting from HIV encephalopathy, or an opportunistic infection or cancer.

This clinical course varies slightly in children with AIDS. Apparently, their incubation time is shorter with a mean of 17 months. Signs and symptoms resemble those in adults, except for findings related to sexually transmitted disease. Children show virtually all of the opportunistic infections observed in adults, with a higher incidence of bacterial infections: otitis media, pneumonias other than *Pneumocystis carinii*, sepsis, chronic salivary gland enlargement, and lymphoid interstitial pneumonia.

Diagnosis

The CDC defines AIDS as an illness characterized by one or more "indicator" diseases coexisting with laboratory evidence of HIV infection and other possible causes for immunosuppression. The CDC's current AIDS surveillance case definition requires laboratory confirmation of HIV infection in persons who have a CD4$^+$ T-lymphocyte count of <200 cells/μL or who have an associated condition or disease.

The most commonly performed tests, antibody tests indicate HIV infection indirectly by revealing HIV antibodies. The recommended protocol requires initial screening of individuals and blood products with an enzyme-linked immunosorbent assay (ELISA) test. A positive ELISA test should be repeated and then confirmed by an alternate method, usually the Western blot or an immunofluorescence assay. How-

(Text continues on page 122.)

Opportunistic diseases associated with AIDS

The following chart describes some common infections associated with acquired immunodeficiency syndrome (AIDS), their characteristic signs and symptoms, and their treatments.

INFECTION	SIGNS AND SYMPTOMS	TREATMENT
Bacterial		
Tuberculosis A disease caused by *Mycobacterium tuberculosis*, an aerobic, acid-fast bacillus spread through inhalation of droplet nuclei that are aerosolized by coughing, sneezing, or talking	Fever, weight loss, night sweats, and fatigue, followed by dyspnea, chills, hemoptysis, and chest pain	Isoniazid, rifampin, pyrazinamide, and ethambutol or streptomycin during the first 2 months of therapy, followed by rifampin and isoniazid for a minimum of 9 months and for at least 6 months after culture is negative for bacteria
***Mycobacterium avium* complex** A primary infection acquired by oral ingestion or inhalation; can infect the bone marrow, liver, spleen, GI tract, lymph nodes, lungs, skin, brain, adrenal glands, and kidneys; is chronic and may be both localized and disseminated in its course of infection	Multiple, nonspecific symptoms consistent with systemic illness: fever, fatigue, weight loss, anorexia, night sweats, abdominal pain, and chronic diarrhea. *Physical examination findings:* emaciation, generalized lymphadenopathy, diffuse tenderness, jaundice, and hepatosplenomegaly. *Laboratory findings:* anemia, leukopenia, and thrombocytopenia	Treatment regimens vary and can include two to six drugs. The Centers for Disease Control and Prevention currently recommends that every patient take either azithromycin or clarithromycin. Many experts prefer ethambutol as a second drug. Additional drugs include clofazimine, rifabutin, rifampin, ciprofloxacin, and sometimes amikacin. Isoniazid and pyrazinamide are not useful.
Salmonellosis A disease acquired by ingestion of contaminated food or water but also linked to snake powders, pet turtles, and domestic turkeys; also can be spread by contaminated medications or diagnostic agents, direct fecal-oral transmission (especially during sexual activity), transfusion of contaminated blood products, and inadequately sterilized fiber-optic instruments used in upper GI endoscopic procedures	Nonspecific signs and symptoms, including fever, chills, sweats, weight loss, diarrhea, and anorexia	Although treatment of nontyphoid salmonellosis is usually unnecessary in immunocompetent individuals, it is required in persons with human immunodeficiency virus (HIV). Antibiotic selection depends on drug sensitivities. However, treatment may include co-trimoxazole, amoxicillin, fluoroquinolones, ampicillin, or third-generation cephalosporins.

Opportunistic diseases associated with AIDS *(continued)*

INFECTION	SIGNS AND SYMPTOMS	TREATMENT
Fungal		
Coccidioidomycosis An infectious disease caused by the fungus *Coccidioides immitis*, which grows in soil in arid regions in the southwestern United States, Mexico, Central America, and South America	Influenza-like illness (malaise, fever, backache, headache, cough, arthralgia), periarticular swelling in knees and ankles, meningitis, bony lesions, skin findings, genitourinary (GU) involvement	Fluconazole, itraconazole, amphotericin B
Candidiasis A disease caused by the fungus *Candida albicans* that exists in unicellular forms on teeth, gingivae, and skin and in the oropharynx, vagina, and large intestine; majority of infections endogenous and related to interruption of normal defense mechanisms; possible human-to-human transmission, including congenital transmission in neonates, in whom thrush develops after vaginal delivery	*Thrush, the most prevalent form in HIV-infected individuals:* creamy, curdlike, yellowish patches, surrounded by an erythematous base, found on buccal membrane and tongue surfaces. *Nail infection:* inflammation and tenderness of tissue surrounding the nails or the nail itself. *Vaginitis:* intense pruritus of the vulva and curdlike vaginal discharge	Nystatin suspension and clotrimazole troches for thrush; nystatin suspension or pastilles, clotrimazole troches, or oral ketoconazole, fluconazole, or itraconazole for esophagitis; topical clotrimazole, miconazole, or ketoconazole for cutaneous candidiasis; topical imidazole or oral fluconazole, ketoconazole, or both for candidiasis of nails; topical clotrimazole, miconazole, or oral ketoconazole for vaginitis
Cryptococcosis An infectious disease caused by the fungus *Cryptococcus neoformans.* It can be found in nature; can be aerosolized and inhaled; settles in the lungs, where it can remain dormant or spread to other parts of the body, particularly the central nervous system (CNS); responsible for three forms of infection: pulmonary, CNS, and disseminated; most pulmonary cases found serendipitously	*Pulmonary cryptococcosis:* fever, cough, dyspnea, and pleuritic chest pain. *CNS cryptococcosis:* fever, malaise, headaches, stiff neck, nausea and vomiting, and altered mentation. *Disseminated cryptococcosis:* lymphadenopathy, multi-focal cutaneous lesions. *Other clinical symptoms:* macules, papules, skin lesions, oral lesions, placental infection, myocarditis, prostatic infection, optic neuropathy, rectal abscess, and peripheral and mediastinal lymph node infection	Primary therapy for initial infection: amphotericin B administered I.V. for 6 to 8 weeks; sometimes amphotericin B and flucytosine combination therapy; fluconazole and itraconazole also used

(continued)

Opportunistic diseases associated with AIDS *(continued)*

INFECTION	SIGNS AND SYMPTOMS	TREATMENT
Fungal *(continued)*		
Histoplasmosis A disease caused by the fungus *Histoplasma capsulatum* that exists in nature, is readily airborne, and can reach the bronchioles and alveoli when inhaled	*Most common:* fever, weight loss, hepatomegaly, splenomegaly, and pancytopenia. *Less common:* diarrhea, cerebritis, chorioretinitis, meningitis, oral and cutaneous lesions, and GI mucosal lesions causing bleeding	Drug of choice: amphotericin B, used as lifelong suppressive therapy, not a cure. Itraconazole is under investigation.
Protozoan		
***Pneumocystis carinii* pneumonia** Pneumonia caused by *Pneumocystis carinii*. This disease also has properties of fungal infection, exists in human lungs, and is transmitted by airborne exposure; the most common life-threatening opportunistic infection in individuals with AIDS	Fever, fatigue, and weight loss for several weeks to months before respiratory symptoms develop. *Respiratory symptoms:* dyspnea, usually noted initially on exertion, later at rest; and cough, usually starting out dry and nonproductive and later becoming productive	Co-trimoxazole orally or I.V. (about 20% of AIDS patients are hypersensitive to sulfa drugs), or I.V. pentamidine isethionate (many adverse effects, including permanent diabetes mellitus). *Also used:* dapsone with trimethoprim, clindamycin, primaquine, atovaquone, or corticosteroids. *Prophylaxis following treatment:* co-trimoxazole, aerosolized pentamidine isethionate or dapsone
Cryptosporidiosis An intestinal infection by the protozoan *Cryptosporidium;* transmitted by person-to-person contact, water, food contaminants, and airborne exposure; most common site: small intestine	Profuse watery diarrhea, abdominal cramping, flatulence, weight loss, anorexia, malaise, fever, nausea, vomiting, and myalgia	No effective therapy. Most medical therapy is palliative and directed toward symptom control, focusing on fluid replacement, occasionally total parenteral nutrition, correction of electrolyte imbalances, and analgesic, antidiarrheal, and antiperistaltic agents. Paromomycin, spiramycin, and eflornithine are used.
Toxoplasmosis A disease caused in humans by *Toxoplasma gondii,* an obligate protozoan; major means of transmission through ingestion of undercooked meats and vegetables containing oocysts; causes focal or diffuse meningoencephalitis with cellular necrosis and progresses unchecked to the lungs, heart, and skeletal muscle	Localized neurologic deficits, fever, headache, altered mental status, and seizures	Sulfadiazine or clindamycin with pyrimethamine (however, about 20% of AIDS patients are hypersensitive to sulfa drugs); folinic acid to prevent marrow toxicity from pyrimethamine

Opportunistic diseases associated with AIDS *(continued)*

INFECTION	SIGNS AND SYMPTOMS	TREATMENT
Protozoan *(continued)*		
Coccidiosis A disease caused by coccidian protozoan parasite *Isospora hominis* or *I. belli*; after ingestion, infects the small intestine and results in malabsorption and diarrhea	Watery, nonbloody diarrhea; crampy abdominal pain; nausea; anorexia; weight loss; weakness; occasional vomiting; and a low-grade fever	Co-trimoxazole for 10 days
Viral		
Herpes simplex virus (HSV) Chronic infection caused by a herpesvirus; often a reactivation of an earlier herpes infection	Red, blisterlike lesions occurring in oral, anal, and genital areas; may also be found on the esophageal and tracheobronchial mucosa in AIDS patients; pain, bleeding, and discharge	Acyclovir is the primary therapy for HSV and is available in I.V., oral, and topical preparations. Vidarabine or foscarnet is used in acyclovir-resistant HSV.
Cytomegalovirus (CMV) A viral infection of the herpesvirus that may result in serious, widespread infection in AIDS patients; most common sites: lungs, adrenal glands, eyes, CNS, GI tract, male GU tract, and blood	Unexplained fever, malaise, GI ulcers, diarrhea, weight loss, swollen lymph nodes, hepatomegaly, splenomegaly, blurred vision, floaters, dyspnea (especially on exertion), and dry, nonproductive cough; vision changes leading to blindness not uncommon in patients with ocular infection	Foscarnet is the drug of choice for CMV retinitis because it lacks the hematologic toxicity of the previous standard, ganciclovir, and has shown some anti-HIV properties.
Progressive multifocal leukoencephalopathy (PML) Progressive demyelinating disorder caused by hyperactivation of a papovavirus that leads to gradual brain degeneration	Progressive dementia, memory loss, headache, confusion, and weakness. Possible other neurologic complications, such as seizures	No form of therapy for PML has been effective, but attempted therapies include prednisone, acyclovir, and adenine arabinoside administered both I.V. and intrathecally.
Herpes zoster A disease also known as acute posterior ganglionitis, shingles, zona, and zoster; acute infection caused by reactivation of the chickenpox virus	Small clusters of painful, reddened papules that follow the route of inflamed nerves; may be disseminated, involving two or more dermatomes	Herpes zoster is most often treated with oral acyclovir capsules until healed. Treatment may have to continue at lower doses indefinitely to prevent recurrence. I.V. acyclovir is effective in disseminated varicella zoster lesions in some patients. Medications may relieve pain associated with the infection and postherpetic neuropathies.

(continued)

Opportunistic diseases associated with AIDS *(continued)*

INFECTION	SIGNS AND SYMPTOMS	TREATMENT
Neoplasms		
Kaposi's sarcoma A generalized disease with characteristic lesions involving all skin surfaces, including the face (tip of the nose, eyelids), head, upper and lower limbs, soles of the feet, palms of the hands, conjunctivae, sclerae, pharynx, larynx, trachea, hard palate, stomach, liver, small and large intestines, and glans penis	Manifested cutaneously and subcutaneously; usually painless, nonpruritic tumor nodules that are pigmented and violaceous (red to blue), nonblanching and palpable; patchy lesions appearing early and possibly mistaken for bruises, purpura, or diffuse cutaneous hemorrhages	Treatment isn't indicated for all individuals. Indications include cosmetically offensive, painful, or obstructive lesions or rapidly progressing disease. Systemic chemotherapy using single or multiple drugs may be given to alleviate symptoms. Radiation therapy may be used to treat lesions. Intralesional therapy with vinblastine may be given for cosmetic purposes to treat small cutaneous lesions, and laser therapy and cryotherapy to treat small isolated lesions. Interferon alfa-2a and interferon alfa-2b are also used.
Malignant lymphomas Immune system cancer in which lymph tissue cells begin growing abnormally and spread to other organs; incidence in persons with AIDS: about 4% to 10%; diagnosed in HIV-infected individuals as widespread disease involving extranodal sites, most commonly in the GI tract, CNS, bone marrow, and liver	Unexplained fever, night sweats, or weight loss greater than 10% of patient's total body weight; signs and symptoms often confined to one body system: CNS (confusion, lethargy, and memory loss) or GI tract (pain, obstruction, changes in bowel habits, bleeding, and fever)	Individualized therapy; modified combination of methotrexate, bleomycin, doxorubicin, cyclophosphamide, vincristine, and dexamethasone; radiation therapy, not chemotherapy, to treat primary CNS lymphoma
Cervical neoplasm Emerging as a significant opportunistic complication of HIV infection as more women become infected with HIV and live longer with illness because of antiretroviral prophylaxis and treatment	*Possible indicators of early invasive disease:* abnormal vaginal bleeding, persistent vaginal discharge, or postcoital pain and bleeding. *Possible indicators of advanced disease:* pelvic pain, vaginal leakage of urine and feces from a fistula, anorexia, weight loss, and fatigue	Treatment tailored to disease stage. Preinvasive lesions: possible total excisional biopsy, cryosurgery, laser destruction, conization (and frequent Papanicolaou test follow-up); rarely, hysterectomy. Invasive squamous cell carcinoma: possible radical hysterectomy and radiation therapy

ever, antibody testing is not always reliable. Because the body takes a variable amount of time to produce a detectable level of antibodies, a "window," varying from a few weeks to as long as 35 months, allows an HIV infected person to test negative for HIV antibodies. Antibody tests are also unreliable in neonates because transferred maternal antibodies persist for 6 to 10 months. To overcome these problems, direct testing can detect HIV. Direct tests include antigen tests (p24 antigen), HIV cultures, nucleic acid probes of peripheral blood lymphocytes, and the polymerase chain reaction.

Additional tests to support the diagnosis and help evaluate the severity of immunosuppression include $CD4^+$ and $CD8^+$ T-lymphocyte subset counts, erythrocyte sedimentation rate (ESR), complete blood cell count, serum $beta_2$-microglobulin, p24 antigen, neopterin levels, and anergy testing. Since many opportunistic infections in AIDS patients are reactivations of previous infections, patients are also tested for syphilis, hepatitis B, tuberculosis, toxoplasmosis and, in some areas, histoplasmosis.

Treatment

No cure has yet been found for AIDS; however, at least three beneficial forms of treatment are available for HIV disease. Several antiretroviral treatments are designed to inhibit or inactivate the HIV virus. Immunomodulatory agents are designed to boost the weakened immune system. Anti-infective and anti-neoplastic agents combat opportunistic infections and associated malignancies; some are used prophylactically to help patients resist opportunistic infections. Current treatment protocols combine two or more agents to gain the maximum benefit with the fewest adverse reactions. Combination therapy also helps inhibit the production of resistant, mutant strains. Supportive treatments help maintain nutritional status and relieve pain and other physical and psychological symptoms.

Many pathogens in AIDS respond to anti-infective drugs but tend to recur after treatment ends. For this reason, most patients need continuous anti-infective treatment, presumably for life or until the drug is no longer tolerated or effective.

Zidovudine slows the progression of HIV infection, decreases opportunistic infections, and prolongs survival. However, it often produces serious adverse reactions and toxicities. The current recommendation is to take 100 mg of zidovudine every 4 hours for a total daily dose of 600 mg, or 500 mg if the patient does not want to interrupt sleep. Didanosine (DDI) may be recommended for patients who cannot tolerate, or who no longer respond to, zidovudine therapy. Zalcitabine (DDC) is used in combination with zidovudine in advanced AIDS to enhance the return of CD4$^+$ T-lymphocyte levels.

Special considerations

Advise health care workers and the public to use precautions in all situations that risk exposure to blood, bodily fluids, and secretions. Practicing universal precautions can prevent inadvertent transmission of AIDS, hepatitis B, and other infectious diseases that are transmitted by similar routes.

Chronic mucocutaneous candidiasis

Also called moniliasis, chronic mucocutaneous candidiasis most commonly develops during the patient's first year of life but occasionally may occur as late as his twenties. Affecting males and females, it's characterized by repeated infection with *Candida albicans* that may result from an inherited defect in cell-mediated (T-cell) immunity. (Humoral immunity, mediated by B cells, is intact and gives a normal antibody response to *C. albicans*.) In some patients, an autoimmune response affecting the endocrine system may induce various endocrinopathies.

Despite chronic candidiasis, these patients rarely die of systemic infection. Instead, they usually die of hepatic or endocrine failure. Prognosis for chronic mucocutaneous candidiasis depends on the severity of the associated endocrinopathy. Indeed, patients with associated endocrinopathy rarely live beyond their thirties.

Causes

Although no characteristic immunologic defects have been identified in this infection, many patients are anergic to various antigens or to *Candida* alone. In some patients, anergy may result from deficient migration inhibition factor, a mediator normally produced by lymphocytes.

Signs and symptoms

Chronic candidal infections can affect the skin, mucous membranes, nails, and vagina, usually causing large, circular lesions. These infections rarely produce systemic symptoms, but in late stages may be associated with recurrent respiratory tract infections. Other associated conditions include severe viral infections that may precede the onset of endocrinopathy and, sometimes, hepatitis. Involvement of the mouth, nose, and palate may cause speech and eating difficulties.

Symptoms of endocrinopathy are peculiar to the organ involved. Tetany and hypocalcemia are most common and are associated with hypoparathyroidism. Addison's disease, hypothyroidism, diabetes, and pernicious anemia are also connected with chronic mucocutaneous candidiasis. Psychiatric disorders are likely because of disfigurement and multiple endocrine aberrations.

Diagnosis

Laboratory findings usually show a normal circulating T-cell count, although it may be decreased. Most patients don't have delayed hypersensitivity skin tests to *Candida,* even during the infectious stage. Migration inhibiting factor that indicates the presence of activated T cells may not respond to *Candida.*

Nonimmunologic abnormalities result from endocrinopathy and may include hypocalcemia, abnormal hepatic function studies, hyperglycemia, iron deficiency, and abnormal vitamin B_{12} absorption (pernicious anemia). Diagnosis must rule out other immunodeficiency disorders associated with chronic *Candida* infection, especially DiGeorge's syndrome, ataxia-telangiectasia, and severe combined immunodeficiency disease, all of which produce severe immunologic defects. After diagnosis, the patient needs evaluation of adrenal, pituitary, thyroid, gonadal, pancreatic, and parathyroid functions, with careful follow-up. The disease is progressive, and most patients eventually develop endocrinopathy.

Treatment

Treatment aims to control infection but isn't always successful. Topical antifungal agents are often ineffective against chronic mucocutaneous candidiasis. Miconazole and nystatin are sometimes useful, but ultimately fail to control this infection.

Systemic infections may not be fatal, but they're serious enough to warrant vigorous treatment. Oral ketaconazole and injected thymosin and levamisole have had some positive effect. Oral or I.M. iron replacement may also be necessary.

Treatment may also include plastic surgery, when possible, and counseling to help patients cope with their disfigurement.

Special
considerations

Teach the patient about the progressive manifestations of the disease and emphasize the importance of seeing an endocrinologist for regular checkups.

Chronic fatigue and immune dysfunction syndrome

Also known as chronic fatigue syndrome, chronic Epstein-Barr virus (EBV), myalgic encephalomyelitis, and "yuppie flu," chronic fatigue and immune dysfunction syndrome is a recently recognized illness that is typically marked by debilitating fatigue, neurologic abnormalities, and persistent symptoms that suggest chronic mononucleosis. It commonly occurs in adults under age 45, primarily in women.

Causes

The syndrome's cause is unknown but researchers suspect human herpesvirus-6 or other herpesviruses, enteroviruses, or retroviruses. Rising levels of antibodies to EBV, once thought to implicate EBV infection as the cause of the syndrome, are now considered a result of it. Chronic fatigue and immune dysfunction syndrome may be associated with a reaction to viral illness that is complicated by dysfunctional immune response and by other factors that may include sex, age, genetic disposition, previous illness, stress, and environment.

Signs and
symptoms

The syndrome's characteristic symptom is prolonged, often overwhelming fatigue that is commonly associated with a varying complex of other symptoms. To aid identification of the disease, the Centers for Disease Control and Prevention (CDC) uses a "working case definition" to group symptoms

CDC criteria for diagnosing chronic fatigue and immune dysfunction syndrome

To meet the Centers for Disease Control and Prevention (CDC)'s case definition of chronic fatigue and immune dysfunction syndrome, a patient must fulfill two major criteria. In addition, he must meet 8 of 11 symptom criteria or the combination of 6 symptom criteria and 2 of 3 physical criteria.

Major criteria
• New onset of persistent or relapsing debilitating fatigue in a person without a history of similar symptoms. The fatigue doesn't resolve with bed rest and is severe enough to reduce or impair average daily activity by 50% for 6 months.
• Exclusion of other disorders after evaluation through history, physical examination, and laboratory findings.

Symptom criteria
The symptom criteria include the initial development of the main symptom complex over a few hours or days and 10 other symptoms.

• Profound or prolonged fatigue, especially after exercise levels that would have been easily tolerated before
• Low-grade fever
• Painful lymph nodes
• Muscle weakness
• Sleep disturbances (insomnia or hypersomnia)
• Headaches of a new type, severity, or pattern
• Migratory arthralgia without joint swelling or redness
• Photophobia, forgetfulness, irritability, confusion, depression, transient visual scotomata, difficulty thinking, and inability to concentrate.

Physical criteria
These criteria must be recorded on at least two occasions, at least 1 month apart.
• Low-grade fever
• Nonexudative pharyngitis
• Palpable or tender nodes

---

and severity. (See *CDC criteria for diagnosing chronic fatigue and immune dysfunction syndrome.*)

Diagnosis

No single test unequivocally confirms the syndrome's presence. Therefore, diagnosis rests on the patient's history and the CDC's criteria. However, because these criteria may not include all forms of the syndrome and are based on symptoms that can result from other diseases, diagnosis is difficult and uncertain.

Treatment

No treatment is known to cure the syndrome. Experimental treatments include the antiviral acyclovir and selected immunomodulating agents such as I.V. gamma globulin, ampligen, transfer factor, and others. Treatment of symptoms may include tricyclic antidepressants (doxepin), histamine$_2$-

blocking agents (cimetidine), and antianxiety agents (alprazolam). In some patients, avoidance of environmental irritants and certain foods may help to relieve symptoms.

Special
considerations

Because affected patients may benefit from the support of others who have the syndrome, suggest the Chronic Fatigue and Immune Dysfunction Syndrome Association for information and referral to local support groups. Patients may also benefit from psychological counseling.

Immunodeficiency with eczema and thrombocytopenia

Known as Wiskott-Aldrich syndrome, this X-linked recessive immunodeficiency affects both B-cell and T-cell function. Its clinical features include thrombocytopenia with severe bleeding, eczema, recurrent infection, and an increased risk of lymphoid cancer. The prognosis is poor. This syndrome causes early death (average life span is 4 years; rarely do affected children survive into their teens), usually from massive bleeding during infancy or from cancer or severe infection in early childhood.

Causes

Because Wiskott-Aldrich syndrome results from an X-linked recessive trait, it affects only males. Children with this genetic defect are born with a normal thymus gland and normal plasma cells and lymphoid tissues. But an inherited defect in both B-cell and T-cell function compromises the child's immune system response and increases his vulnerability to infection. These children also have a metabolic defect in platelet synthesis that causes them to produce only small, short-lived platelets, resulting in thrombocytopenia.

Signs and
symptoms

Characteristically, newborns with Wiskott-Aldrich syndrome develop bloody stools, bleeding from a circumcision site, petechiae, and purpura as a result of thrombocytopenia. As these infants get older, thrombocytopenia subsides. But beginning at about 6 months, they typically develop recurrent systemic infections, such as chronic pneumonia, sinusitis, otitis media, and herpes simplex of the skin and eyes (which may cause keratitis and vision loss), with hepatospleno-megaly. Usually, *Streptococcus pneumoniae,* meningococci, and *Haemophilus influenzae* are the infecting organisms. At about 1 year, eczema develops and becomes progressively more severe. Skin is easily infected because of persistent scratching. These children are also highly vulnerable to certain cancers, especially leukemia and lymphoma.

Diagnosis

The most important clues to diagnosis of Wiskott-Aldrich syndrome are thrombocytopenia (demonstrated by coagulation tests showing a platelet count below 100,000/mm^3 and prolonged bleeding time) and bleeding disorders at birth. Laboratory tests may show normal or elevated immunoglobulin E (IgE) and IgA levels, decreased IgM levels, normal IgG levels, and low levels or absence of isohemagglutinins. In newborns, T-cell immunity may be normal, but it gradually declines with age.

Treatment

Treatment aims to limit bleeding through the use of fresh, cross-matched platelet transfusions; to prevent or control infection with prophylactic or early and aggressive antibiotic therapy as appropriate; to supply passive immunity with immune globulin infusion; and to control eczema with topical corticosteroids. (Systemic corticosteroids are contraindicated because they further compromise immunity.) An antipruritic may relieve itching.

Treatment with transfer factor has had limited success. However, bone marrow transplantation has been remarkably successful in some patients.

Special
considerations

• Physical and psychological support and patient teaching can help these children and their families cope with this disorder. As soon as the child is old enough, begin teaching him about his disease and his limitations.
• Teach parents of an affected child to watch him for signs of bleeding, such as easy bruising, bloody stools, swollen joints, and tenderness in the trunk area. Help them plan their child's activity levels to ensure normal development. Al-

though the child must avoid contact sports, he is allowed to ride a bike (while wearing protective gear) and swim.
• Before giving platelet transfusions, establish the child's baseline platelet count. Be sure to check the platelet count often during therapy; each platelet unit transfused should raise the count by 10,000/mm^3.
• Instruct parents to observe the child for signs of infection, such as fever, coldlike symptoms, or drainage and redness around any superficial wound, and to report such signs promptly. Emphasize the importance of meticulous mouth and skin care (including careful cleaning of all skin wounds, no matter how superficial), good nutrition, and adequate hydration. Stress the need to avoid exposing the child to crowds or to persons who have active infections.
• As appropriate, arrange for the parents of children with Wiskott-Aldrich syndrome to receive genetic counseling to answer any questions they may have about the potential vulnerability of their future offspring.

Ataxia-telangiectasia

Inherited as an autosomal recessive disorder, ataxia-telangiectasia is characterized by progressively severe ataxia; telangiectasia, particularly of the face, earlobes, and conjunctivae; and chronic, recurrent sinopulmonary infections that may reflect both humoral (B-cell) and cell-mediated (T-cell) immunodeficiencies. At one time, ataxia-telangiectasia was considered a neurologic disease, because its dominant sign is cerebellar ataxia. It's now known to have associated endocrine and vascular aspects. Ataxia usually appears within 2 years after birth, but may develop as late as age 9. The degree of immunodeficiency determines the rate of deterioration. Some patients die within several years; others survive until their thirties. Severe abnormalities cause rapid clinical deterioration and premature death due to overwhelming sinopulmonary infection or cancer.

Causes

In this autosomal recessive disorder, immunodeficiency may result from defective embryonic development of the mesoderm, hormone deficiency, or defective deoxyribonucleic acid repair.

Signs and symptoms

The earliest and most dominant signs of cerebellar ataxia usually develop by the time the infant begins to use his motor skills. They typically include continual, involuntary, spastic (choreoathetoid) movements; nystagmus; extrapyramidal symptoms (pseudoparkinsonism, motor restlessness, dystonia); and posterior column signs (decreased arm movements, purposeless tremors, and unsteady gait with leaning forward to maintain balance).

The associated telangiectasia usually appears later and may not develop until age 9, appearing first as a vascular lesion on the sclera and later on the bridge or side of the nose, the ear, or the antecubital or popliteal areas.

Approximately 80% of affected children develop recurrent or chronic respiratory infections because of immunoglobulin A (IgA) deficiency early in life, but some may be symptom-free for 10 years or more. These children are unusually vulnerable to lymphomas, particularly lymphosarcomas and lymphoreticular cancers, and may also develop leukemia, adenocarcinoma, dysgerminoma, or medulloblastoma. They may fail to develop secondary sex characteristics during puberty and eventually may become mentally retarded.

Rarely, a patient shows signs of progeria: premature graying of hair, senile keratoses, and vitiligo.

Diagnosis

If a patient has the complete syndrome (ataxia, telangiectasia, and recurrent sinopulmonary infection), the diagnosis can be made on these clinical facts alone. However, the complete syndrome may not be apparent, and ataxia may be the only symptom for 6 years or longer. Therefore, early diagnosis usually depends on immunologic tests. A patient with ataxia-telangiectasia usually shows the following:
• selective absence of IgA (in 60% to 80%) or deficient IgA and IgE
• normal B-cell count but diminished antibody responses
• absence of Hassall's corpuscles on examination of thymic tissue

• high serum levels of oncofetal proteins
• decreased T-cell count.

Physical examination reveals degenerative neurologic changes; these can also be demonstrated by computed tomography scan, magnetic resonance imaging, and pneumoencephalography.

Treatment

No treatment is yet available to stop progression of ataxia-telangiectasia. However, prophylactic or early and aggressive therapy with broad-spectrum antibiotics is essential to prevent or control recurrent infections.

Immune globulin infusion or injection can passively replace missing antibodies in an IgG-deficient patient and may also help prevent infection. (This treatment may not help an IgA-deficient patient, however.) The effectiveness of other forms of immunotherapy—such as fetal thymus transplant or histocompatible bone marrow transplant—is unproven.

Special considerations

• To help parents protect their child from infections, advise them to avoid crowds and persons who have infections, and teach them to recognize early signs of infection.
• Teach parents physical therapy and postural drainage techniques if their child has chronic bronchial infections.
• As always, stress proper nutrition and adequate hydration.
• Parents of a child with ataxia-telangiectasia may have questions about the vulnerability of their future offspring and may need genetic counseling. They may also need psychological therapy to help them cope with their child's long-term illness and inevitable early death.

Chronic granulomatous disease

In chronic granulomatous disease (CGD), abnormal neutrophil metabolism impairs phagocytosis—one of the body's chief defense mechanisms—resulting in increased susceptibility to low-virulent or nonpathogenic organisms, such as *Staphylococcus epidermidis, Escherichia coli, Aspergillus,* and *Nocardia.* Phagocytes attracted to sites of infection can engulf these invading organisms but are unable to destroy them. Patients with CGD may develop granulomatous inflammation, which leads to ischemic tissue damage.

Causes

CGD is usually inherited as an X-linked trait, although a variant form – probably autosomal recessive – also exists. The genetic defect may be linked to deficiency of the enzyme nicotinamide adenine dinucleotide (NADH), nicotinamide adenine dinucleotide phosphate oxidase (NADPH), or NADH reductase.

Signs and symptoms

Usually, the patient with CGD displays signs and symptoms by age 2, associated with infections of the skin, lymph nodes, lung, liver, and bone. Skin infection is characterized by small, well-localized areas of tenderness. Seborrheic dermatitis of the scalp and axilla is also common. Lymph node infection typically causes marked lymphadenopathy with draining lymph nodes and hepatosplenomegaly. Many patients develop liver abscess, which may be recurrent and multiple; abdominal tenderness, fever, anorexia, and nausea point to abscess formation. Other common infections include osteomyelitis, which causes localized pain and fever; pneumonia; and gingivitis with severe periodontal disease.

Diagnosis

Clinical features of osteomyelitis, pneumonia, liver abscess, or chronic lymphadenopathy in a young child provide the first clues to diagnosis of CGD. An important tool for confirming this diagnosis is the nitroblue tetrazolium (NBT) test. A clear yellow dye, NBT is normally reduced by neutrophil metabolism, resulting in a color change from yellow to blue. Quantifying this color change estimates the degree of neutrophil metabolism. Patients with CGD show impaired NBT reduction, indicating abnormal neutrophil metabolism. Another test measures the rate of intracellular killing by neutrophils; in CGD, killing is delayed or absent.

Other laboratory values may support the diagnosis or help monitor disease activity. Osteomyelitis typically causes an elevated white blood cell count and erythrocyte sedimentation rate; bone scans help locate infections. Recurrent liver or lung infection may eventually cause abnormal function studies. Cell-mediated and humoral immunity are usually normal in CGD, although some patients have hypergammaglobulinemia.

Treatment

Early, aggressive treatment of infection is the chief goal in caring for a patient with CGD. Areas of suspected infection should be studied through biopsy or culture, with broad-spectrum antibiotics usually started immediately – without waiting for results of cultures. Confirmed abscesses may be drained or surgically removed.

Many patients with CGD receive a combination of I.V. antibiotics, often extended beyond the usual 10- to 14-day course. However, for fungal infections with *Aspergillus* or *Nocardia,* treatment involves amphotericin B in gradually increasing doses to achieve a maximum cumulative dose.

To help treat life-threatening or antibiotic-resistant infection or to help localize infection, the patient may receive granulocyte transfusions – usually once daily until the crisis has passed.

Interferon is an experimental but promising treatment in CGD.

Special considerations

• Provide meticulous wound care after treatment of abscesses, including irrigation or packing.
• During I.V. drug therapy, monitor vital signs frequently and rotate the I.V. site every 48 to 72 hours.
• During granulocyte transfusions, watch for fever and chills (these effects can sometimes be prevented by premedication with acetaminophen).
• Transfusions should not be given for 6 hours before or after amphotericin B to avoid severe pulmonary edema and possibly respiratory arrest.
• If prophylactic antibiotics are ordered, teach the patient and his family how to administer them properly and how to recognize adverse effects.
• Advise the patient or his family to promptly report any signs or symptoms of infection.
• Stress the importance of good nutrition and hygiene, especially meticulous skin and mouth care.
• During hospitalizations, encourage the patient to continue his activities of daily living as much as possible.
• Try to arrange for a tutor to help the child keep up with his schoolwork.

Chédiak-Higashi syndrome

Chédiak-Higashi syndrome (CHS) is characterized by morphologic changes in granulocytes that impair their ability to respond to chemotaxis and to digest or "kill" invading organisms. This rare syndrome has been documented in about 100 cases worldwide. It also affects certain animals, including cows, mice, whales, tigers, and minks. Partial albinism is typically associated with CHS.

Causes

CHS is transmitted as an autosomal recessive trait. In many cases, it seems linked to consanguinity. The genetic defect is expressed by morphologic changes in the granulocytes, which contain giant granules with abnormal lysosomal enzymes. These abnormal granulocytes display delayed chemotaxis and impaired intracellular digestion of organisms, both of which diminish the inflammatory response.

Signs and symptoms

The child with CHS has recurrent bacterial infections, most commonly caused by *Staphylococcus aureus* but also by streptococci and pneumococci. These infections occur primarily in the skin, subcutaneous tissue, and lungs and may be accompanied by fever, thrombocytopenia, neutropenia, and hepatosplenomegaly.

Partial albinism in CHS involves the ocular fundi, skin, and hair, which has a characteristic silvery sheen. Most patients also have significant photophobia. Progressive motor and sensory neuropathy may eventually cause debilitation and inability to walk or perform activities of daily living. Patients who survive recurrent bouts of infection commonly develop marked proliferation of granulocytes or lymphocytes, resembling lymphoreticular malignancy. These cells infiltrate the liver, spleen, and bone marrow, causing progressively severe hepatosplenomegaly, thrombocytopenia, neutropenia, and anemia. Eventually, this cellular proliferation is fatal.

Diagnosis

Diagnosis of CHS rests on detection of characteristic morphologic changes in granulocytes on a peripheral smear.

Functional studies confirm delayed chemotaxis of granulocytes and impaired intracellular digestion of organisms.

Treatment

When prevention of infection fails, the next-best step is early detection and vigorous treatment of infection with antimicrobials and surgical drainage if indicated.

In a few patients, large doses of vitamin C (ascorbic acid) have helped enhance chemotaxis of abnormal granulocytes, although without associated clinical improvement.

Special considerations

• Provide meticulous skin care to maintain skin integrity and prevent infection.
• Teach the patient and his family how to prevent and recognize infection, especially in areas of decreased sensation.
• After surgical drainage of infection, provide diligent wound care. Irrigate draining or open wounds and change sterile dressings frequently.
• Administer antimicrobials and monitor the patient for adverse reactions to drugs. Also check the I.V. site frequently.
• Suggest sunglasses or a visor, or both, to minimize discomfort from photophobia. Also teach the patient how to avoid injury associated with decreased sensation or motor coordination.
• Offer emotional support to help the patient and his family cope with this difficult disorder and maintain as normal a lifestyle as possible.

Severe combined immunodeficiency disease

In severe combined immunodeficiency disease (SCID), both cell-mediated (T-cell) and humoral (B-cell) immunity are deficient or absent, resulting in susceptibility to infection from all classes of microorganisms during infancy. At least three types of SCID exist: reticular dysgenesis, the most severe type, in which the hematopoietic stem cell fails to differentiate into lymphocytes and granulocytes; Swiss-type agammaglobuli-nemia, in which the hematopoietic stem cell fails to differentiate into lymphocytes alone; and enzyme deficiency, such as adenosine deaminase (ADA) deficiency, in which the buildup of toxic products in the lymphoid tissue causes damage and subsequent dysfunction. SCID affects more males than females; its estimated incidence is 1 in every 100,000 to 500,000 births. Most untreated patients die from infection within 1 year of birth.

Causes

SCID is usually transmitted as an autosomal recessive trait, although it may be X-linked. In most cases, the genetic defect seems associated with failure of the stem cell to differentiate into T and B lymphocytes. Many molecular defects can cause SCID. X-linked SCID is due to a mutation of a subunit of the interleukin-2 (IL-2), IL-4, and IL-7 receptors. Less commonly, it results from an enzyme deficiency.

Signs and symptoms

An extreme susceptibility to infection becomes obvious in the infant with SCID in the first months of life. The infant fails to thrive and develops chronic otitis; sepsis; watery diarrhea (associated with *Salmonella* or *Escherichia coli*); recurrent pulmonary infections (usually caused by *Pseudomonas,* cytomegalovirus, or *Pneumocystis carinii*); persistent oral candidiasis, sometimes with esophageal erosions; and possibly fatal, viral infections (such as chickenpox).

P. carinii pneumonia usually strikes a severely immunodeficient infant in the first 3 to 5 weeks of life. Onset is typically insidious, with gradually worsening cough, low-grade fever, tachypnea, and respiratory distress. A chest X-ray characteristically shows bilateral pulmonary infiltrates.

Diagnosis

Diagnosis is generally made clinically, because most SCID infants suffer recurrent overwhelming infections within 1 year of birth. Some infants are diagnosed after a severe reaction to vaccination.

Defective humoral immunity is difficult to detect before an infant is 5 months old. Before age 5 months, even normal infants have very small amounts of serum immunoglobulin M (IgM) and IgA, and normal IgG levels merely reflect maternal IgG. However, severely diminished or absent T-cell number and function and lymph node biopsy showing absence of lymphocytes can confirm diagnosis of SCID.

Treatment

Treatment aims to restore immune response and prevent infection. Histocompatible bone marrow transplant is the only satisfactory treatment available to correct immunodeficiency. Because bone marrow cells must be matched according to human leukocyte antigen and mixed leukocyte culture, the most common donors are histocompatible siblings. But because bone marrow transplant can produce a potentially fatal graft-versus-host (GVH) reaction, newer methods of bone marrow transplant that eliminate GVH reaction (such as lectin separation and the use of monoclonal antibodies) are being evaluated. (See *Iatrogenic immunodeficiency.*)

Fetal thymus and liver transplants have achieved limited success. Administration of immune globulin may also play a role in treatment. Some SCID infants have received long-term protection by being isolated in a completely sterile environment. However, this approach isn't effective if the infant already has had recurring infections.

Gene therapy is being used for ADA deficiency.

Special considerations

• Constantly monitor the infant for early signs of infection; if infection develops, provide prompt and aggressive drug therapy.
• Watch for adverse effects of any medications given.
• Avoid vaccinations, and give only irradiated blood products if transfusion is necessary.
• Although SCID infants must remain in strict protective isolation, try to provide a stimulating atmosphere to promote growth and development.
• Encourage parents to visit their child often, to hold him, and to bring him toys that can be easily sterilized.
• Explain all procedures, medications, and precautions to the parents.
• Maintain a normal daily and nightly routine, and talk to the child as much as possible. If the parents cannot visit, call them often to report on the infant's condition.
• Because parents will have questions about the vulnerability of their future offspring, refer them for genetic counseling.

Iatrogenic immunodeficiency

Iatrogenic immunodeficiency may be a complicating adverse effect of chemotherapy or other treatment. At times, though, it's the very goal of therapy—for example, to suppress immune-mediated tissue damage in autoimmune disorders or to prevent rejection of an organ transplant.

As explained below, iatrogenic immunodeficiency may be induced by immunosuppressive drugs, radiation therapy, or splenectomy.

Immunosuppressive drug therapy

Immunosuppressive drugs fall into several categories:

• **Cytotoxic drugs.** These drugs kill immunocompetent cells while they're replicating. However, most cytotoxic drugs aren't selective and thus interfere with all rapidly proliferating cells. As a result, they reduce the number of lymphocytes as well as phagocytes. Besides depleting their number, cytotoxic drugs interfere with lymphocyte synthesis and the release of immunoglobulins and lymphokines.

Cyclophosphamide is a potent and frequently used immunosuppressant that initially depletes the number of B cells. This causes suppression of humoral immunity. However, chronic therapy also depletes T cells, suppressing cell-mediated immunity as well. Cyclophosphamide may be used in systemic lupus erythematosus, Wegener's granulomatosis, and other systemic vasculitides, and in certain autoimmune disorders. Because it nonselectively destroys rapidly dividing cells, this drug can cause severe bone marrow suppression with neutropenia, anemia, and thrombocytopenia; gonadal suppression with sterility; alopecia; hemorrhagic cystitis; and nausea, vomiting, and sto-

matitis. It may also increase the risk of lymphoproliferative cancer.

Among other cytotoxic drugs used for immunosuppression are azathioprine, which is frequently used in kidney transplantation, and methotrexate, which is occasionally used in rheumatoid arthritis and other autoimmune disorders.

If the patient is receiving cytotoxic drugs, monitor his white blood cell (WBC) count; if it falls too low, the drug dosage may need to be adjusted. Also monitor urine output and watch for signs of cystitis, especially if the patient is taking cyclophosphamide. Ensure adequate fluid intake (2 liters daily). Give mesna to help prevent hemorrhagic cystitis. Provide antiemetics to relieve nausea and vomiting. Give the patient meticulous oral hygiene and watch for signs of stomatitis.

Teach the patient about the early signs and symptoms of infection. If his WBC count falls too low, granulocyte colony-stimulating factor may be used to boost the count. Suggest wearing a scarf, hat, or wig to hide temporary alopecia. Make sure the male patient understands the risk of sterility; advise sperm banking if appropriate. Young women may take oral contraceptives to minimize ovarian dysfunction and to prevent pregnancy during administration of these potentially teratogenic drugs.

• **Corticosteroids.** These adrenocortical hormones are used to treat immune-mediated disorders because of their potent anti-inflammatory and immunosuppressive effects. Corticosteroids stabilize the vascular membrane, blocking tissue infiltration by neutrophils and monocytes, thus inhibiting inflammation. They also "kidnap" T cells in the bone

(continued)

Iatrogenic immunodeficiency *(continued)*

marrow, causing lymphopenia. Because these drugs aren't cytotoxic, lymphocyte concentration can return to normal within 24 hours after they are withdrawn. Corticosteroids also appear to inhibit immunoglobulin synthesis and to interfere with the binding of immunoglobulin to antigen or to cells with Fc receptors. These drugs have many other effects as well.

The most commonly used oral corticosteroid is prednisone. For long-term therapy, prednisone is best given early in the morning to minimize exogenous suppression of cortisol production and with food or milk to minimize gastric irritation. After the acute phase, it's usually reduced to an alternate-day schedule and then gradually withdrawn to minimize potentially harmful adverse effects. Other corticosteroids used for immunosuppression include hydrocortisone, methylprednisolone, and dexamethasone.

Chronic corticosteroid therapy can cause numerous adverse effects, which are sometimes more harmful than the disease itself. Neurologic adverse effects include euphoria, insomnia, or psychosis; cardiovascular effects include hypertension and edema; and GI effects include gastric irritation, ulcers, and increased appetite with weight gain. Other possible effects are cataracts, hyperglycemia, glucose intolerance, muscle weakness, osteoporosis, delayed wound healing, and increased susceptibility to infection.

During corticosteroid therapy, monitor the patient's blood pressure, weight, and intake and output. Instruct the patient to eat a well-balanced, low-salt diet or to follow his specially prescribed diet to prevent excessive weight gain. Remember that even though the patient is actually more susceptible to infection during therapy, he'll show fewer or less dramatic signs of inflammation than before.

• **Cyclosporine.** A relatively new immunosuppressive drug, cyclosporine selectively suppresses the proliferation and development of helper T cells, resulting in depressed cell-mediated immunity. This drug is used primarily to prevent rejection of kidney, liver, and heart transplants but is also being investigated for use in several other disorders. Significant toxic effects of cyclosporine primarily involve the liver and kidney, so treatment with this drug requires regular evaluation of renal and hepatic function. Some studies also link cyclosporine with increased risk of lymphoma. Adjusting the dose or the duration of therapy helps minimize certain adverse effects.

• **Antilymphocyte serum or antithymocyte globulin.** This anti–T cell antibody reduces T-cell number and function, thus suppressing cell-mediated immunity. It has been used effectively to prevent cell-mediated rejection of tissue grafts or transplants. Usually, antilymphocyte serum or antithymocyte globulin (ATG) is administered immediately before the transplant and continued for some time afterward. Potential adverse effects include anaphylaxis and serum sickness. Occurring 1 to 2 weeks after injection of ATG, serum sickness is characterized by fever, malaise, rash, arthralgia, and occasionally glomerulonephritis or vasculitis. It presumably results from the deposition of immune complexes throughout the body.

Radiation therapy
Because irradiation is cytotoxic to proliferating and intermitotic cells, including most lymphocytes, radiation therapy

Iatrogenic immunodeficiency (continued)

may induce profound lymphopenia, resulting in immunosuppression. Radiation of all major lymph node areas — a procedure known as total nodal irradiation — is used to treat certain disorders such as Hodgkin's disease. Its effectiveness in severe rheumatoid arthritis, lupus nephritis, and prevention of kidney transplant rejection is still under investigation.

Splenectomy
After splenectomy, the patient has increased susceptibility to infection, especially with pyogenic bacteria such as *Streptococcus pneumoniae*. This risk of infection is even greater when the patient is very young or has an underlying reticuloendothelial disorder. The incidence of fulminant, rapidly fatal bacteremia is especially high in splenectomized patients and often follows trauma. These patients should receive Pneumovax immunization for prophylaxis and be warned to avoid exposure to infection and trauma.

• Refer parents, siblings, and other close family members for psychological and spiritual support to help them cope with the child's inevitable long-term illness and early death. They may also need a social service referral for assistance in coping with the financial burden of the child's long-term hospitalization.

Complement deficiencies

Complement is a series of circulating enzymatic serum proteins with nine functional components (C), labeled C1 through C9. (The first four complement components are numbered out of sequence because they were numbered in the order of their discovery. These are C1, C4, C2, and C3. The remaining five, however, are numbered sequentially.)

When immunoglobulin G (IgG) or IgM reacts with antigens as part of an immune response, it activates C1, which then combines with C4, initiating the classic complement pathway, or cascade. (An alternative complement pathway involves the direct activation of C3 by the serum protein properdin, bypassing the initial components [C1, C4, C2] of the classic pathway.) Complement then combines with the antigen-antibody complex and undergoes a sequence of reactions that amplifies the immune response against the antigen. This complex process is called complement fixation.

Complement deficiency or dysfunction may increase susceptibility to infection and also seems related to certain autoimmune disorders. Theoretically, any complement component may be deficient or dysfunctional, and many such disorders are under investigation.

Primary complement deficiencies are rare. The most common ones are C2, C4, C6, and C8 deficiencies and C5 familial dysfunction. More common secondary complement abnormalities have been confirmed in patients with lupus erythematosus, in some with dermatomyositis, and in one with scleroderma. (These secondary complement abnormalities were also confirmed in the family of the patient with scleroderma.) In a few patients with gonococcal and meningococcal infections, common secondary complement abnormalities were also confirmed. The prognosis varies with the abnormality and the severity of associated diseases.

Causes

Primary complement deficiencies are inherited as autosomal recessive traits, except for deficiency of C1 esterase inhibitor, which is autosomal dominant. Secondary deficiencies may follow complement-fixing (complement-consuming) immunologic reactions, such as drug-induced serum sickness, acute streptococcal glomerulonephritis, and acute, active systemic lupus erythematosus.

Signs and symptoms

Clinical effects vary with the specific deficiency. C2 and C3 deficiencies and C5 familial dysfunction increase susceptibility to bacterial infection. This increased susceptibility may involve several body systems simultaneously. C2 and C4 deficiencies are also associated with collagen vascular disease, such as lupus erythematosus, and with chronic renal failure. C5 dysfunction, a familial defect in infants, causes failure to thrive, diarrhea, and seborrheic dermatitis. C1 esterase inhibitor deficiency (hereditary angioedema) may cause periodic swelling in the face, hands, abdomen, or throat, with potentially fatal laryngeal edema.

Diagnosis

Diagnosis of a complement deficiency is difficult and requires careful interpretation of both clinical features and laboratory results. Total serum complement level is low in various complement deficiencies. In addition, specific assays may be done to confirm deficiency of specific complement components. For example, detection of complement components and IgG by immunofluorescent examination of glomerular tissues in glomerulonephritis strongly suggests complement deficiency.

Treatment

Primary complement deficiencies have no known cure. Associated infection, collagen vascular disease, or renal disease requires prompt, appropriate treatment.

Transfusion of fresh frozen plasma to provide replacement of complement components is one treatment, a controversial one because replacement therapy doesn't cure complement deficiencies and any beneficial effects are transient. Bone marrow transplant may also be helpful. But this treatment can cause a potentially fatal graft-versus-host (GVH) reaction. Anabolic steroids, such as danazol, and antifibrinolytic agents are often used to reduce acute swelling in patients with C1 esterase inhibitor deficiency.

Special considerations

• Teach the patient the importance of avoiding infection, how to recognize its early signs and symptoms, and the need for prompt treatment if it occurs. If the patient is a child, make sure his family understands the best ways to avoid and treat infection.
• Following bone marrow transplantation, make sure you monitor the patient closely for signs of either transfusion reaction or GVH reaction.
• Meticulous patient care can speed recovery and prevent complications. For example, a patient with renal infection needs careful monitoring of intake and output, tests for serum electrolytes and acid-base balance, and observation for signs of renal failure.
• When caring for a patient with hereditary angioedema, be prepared for emergency management of laryngeal edema; keep airway equipment on hand.

Self-test questions

You can quickly review your comprehension of this chapter on immunodeficiency by answering the following questions. The correct answers to these questions and their rationales appear on pages 156 to 158.

Case history questions

Jimmy Williamson, a 10-month-old infant, has been recently diagnosed with X-linked infantile hypogammaglobulinemia (XLA) after experiencing recurrent bacterial infections and developmental retardation without lymphadenopathy or splenomegaly.

1. In XLA, immunoglobulins are absent or deficient because a mutation in the B-cell protein tyrosine kinase causes:
    a. an absence of B cells from bone marrow and peripheral blood.
    b. failure of B-cell precursors to survive and mature in the bone marrow.
    c. premature death of circulating B cells.
    d. failure of B cells to mature and secrete immunoglobulins.

2. Which absent immunoglobulin does immune globulin primarily replace?
    a. IgG
    b. IgA
    c. Mucosal secretory IgA
    d. IgM

Jonathan Kinsey, age 32, was infected with the human immunodeficiency virus (HIV) Type I. He's quite certain that he was infected by a casual sexual contact during receptive rectal intercourse.

3. Jonathan was definitively diagnosed using the:
    a. ELISA test.
    b. Western blot assay.
    c. immunofluorescence assay.
    d. antigen test.

4. Which of the following initial adverse effects would most likely have prompted Jonathan to seek testing?
    a. Persistent, generalized lymphadenopathy
    b. Neurologic symptoms
    c. Mononucleosis-like syndrome
    d. Candidal infection

5. To slow progression of HIV infection, Jonathan would initially receive:
    a. didanosine.
    b. zalcitabine.
    c. zidovudine.
    d. pentamidine.

6. AIDS dementia complex occurs because of:
    a. CD4$^+$ T-lymphocyte dysfunction.
    b. direct destruction of neuroglial cells.
    c. direct destruction of CD4$^+$ T cells.
    d. immunosuppression resulting indirectly from CD4$^+$ T-lymphocyte dysfunction.

Additional questions

7. Although the cause of chronic fatigue and immune dysfunction syndrome is unknown, researchers currently suspect:
    a. a retrovirus.
    b. the Epstein-Barr virus.
    c. a reaction to a bacterial illness.
    d. an inherited T-cell defect.

8. Which of the following opportunistic infections, commonly associated with acquired immunodeficiency syndrome, usually strikes infants with severe combined immunodeficiency in the first 3 to 5 weeks of their lives?
    a. Histoplasmosis
    b. Cytomegalovirus infection
    c. *Pneumocystis carinii* pneumonia
    d. Candidal infection

9. In complement deficiencies, deficiencies of C2 and C4 are associated with:
    a. increased susceptibility to bacterial infections.
    b. failure to thrive, diarrhea, and seborrheic dermatitis.

    c. hereditary angioedema.

    d. collagen vascular disease and chronic renal failure.

10. When a patient has DiGeorge's syndrome, his initial treatment will focus on:

    a. correction of cardiac anomalies.

    b. management of hypocalcemia.

    c. fetal thymus transplant.

    d. repair of facial anomalies.

Selected References
and Self-Test Answers and Rationales

Selected References

Ayuso-Peralta, L., et al. "Progressive Multifocal Leukoencepha-lopathy in HIV Infection Presenting as Balint's Syndrome," *Neurology* 44(7):1339-40, July 1994.

Berger, J.R., and Levy, R.M. "The Neurologic Complications of Human Immunodeficiency Virus Infection," *Medical Clinics of North America* 77(1):1-23, January 1993.

Bousquet, J., and Michel, F.B. *Journal of Allergy and Clinical Immunology* 94(1):1-11, July 1994.

Demoly, P., et al. "Cell Proliferation in the Bronchial Mucosa of Asthmatics and Chronic Bronchitics," *American Journal of Respiratory and Critical Care Medicine* 150(1):214-17, July 1994.

Lockwood, C.M., et al. "Long-Term Remission of Intractable Systemic Vasculitis with Monoclonal Antibody Therapy," *Lancet* 341(8861):1620-22, June 26, 1993.

Long, A.F., et al. "Measuring Health Status and Outcomes in Rheumatoid Arthritis within Routine Clinical Practice," *British Journal of Rheumatology* 33(7):682-85, July 1994.

Miller-Blair, D.J., and Robbins, D.L. "Rheumatoid Arthritis: New Science, New Treatment," *Geriatrics* 48(6):28-31, 35-38, June 1993.

Nunn, P., et al. "A Deadly Duo — TB and AIDS," *World Health* (4): 7-9, July-August 1993.

Roitt, I., et al. *Immunology,* 3rd ed. St. Louis: Mosby–Year Book, Inc., 1993.

Rönnelid, J., et al. "Local Anti-Type II Collagen Antibody Production in Rheumatoid Arthritis Synovial Fluid. Evidence for an HLA-DR4-Restricted IgG Response." *Arthritis and Rheumatism* 37(7):1023-29, July 1994.

Schumacher, H.R., Jr., ed. *Primer on the Rheumatic Diseases,* 10th ed. Atlanta: Arthritis Foundation, 1993.

Workman, M.L., et al. *Nursing Care of the Immunocompromised Patient.* Philadelphia: W.B. Saunders Co., 1993.

Self-Test Answers and Rationales

Chapter 1:
Introduction

1. b The thymus participates in the maturation of T lymphocytes (cell-mediated immunity); here, these cells are "educated" to differentiate between self and nonself. In contrast, B lymphocytes (humoral immunity) mature in the bone marrow. The key humoral effector mechanism is the production of immunoglobulins by B cells and the subsequent activation of the complement cascade. The lymph nodes, spleen, liver, and intestinal lymphoid tissue help remove and destroy circulating antigens in the blood and lymphatic system.

2. d T and B lymphocytes have specific surface receptors that respond to antigen molecular shapes (epitopes). The T-cell antigen receptor recognizes an antigen only in association with specific cell surface molecules, known as the major histocompatibility complex (MCH). MCH molecules are polymorphic; that is, they differ among individuals. They form the basis of self versus nonself recognition. In B cells, this antigen receptor is an immunoglobulin (antibody) cell: immunoglobulin D (IgD) or IgM; it is sometimes referred to as a surface immunoglobulin.

3. d One of the most important functions of macrophages is the presentation of antigen to T lymphocytes. Macrophages ingest and process antigen, then deposit it on their own surfaces in association with human leukocyte antigen. T lymphocytes become activated upon recognizing this complex. Macrophages also function in the inflammatory response by producing interleukin-1 (IL-1), which generates fever, and by synthesizing complement proteins and other mediators that produce phagocytic, microbicidal, and tumoricidal effects.

4. c Once C3 is activated in either pathway, activation of the terminal components—C5 to C9—follows. In the classical pathway, binding of IgM or IgG and an antigen forms antigen-antibody complexes that activate the first complement component, C1. This, in turn, activates C4, C2, and C3. In the alternate pathway, activating surfaces, such as bacterial membranes, directly amplify spontaneous cleavage of C3.

5. a As a secretory immunoglobulin, IgA defends external body surfaces and is present in colostrum, saliva, tears, nasal fluids, and respiratory, GI, and genitourinary secretions. IgG, the smallest immunoglobulin, constitutes 75% of the total immunoglobulins and is the major antibacterial and antiviral antibody. IgE, present in trace amounts in serum, is involved in the release of vasoactive amines stored in basophils and mast cell granules. When released, these bioamines cause the allergic effects characteristic of this type of hypersensitivity (erythema, itching, smooth muscle contraction, secretions, and swelling). IgD, present as a monomer in serum in minute amounts, is the predominant antibody found on the surface of B lymphocytes and serves mainly as an antigen receptor. It may function in controlling activation or suppression of lymphocytes.

6. a Interferons act very early to limit spread of viral infections. They also inhibit tumor growth. Mainly, they determine how well tissue cells interact with cytotoxic cells and lymphocytes. Colony-stimulating factors mainly function as hematopoietic growth factors, guiding the division and differentiation of bone marrow stem cells. They also influence the function of mature lymphocytes, monocytes, macrophages, and neutrophils. Tumor necrosis factors are thought to play an important role in mediating inflammation and cytotoxic reactions (along with IL-1, IL-6, and IL-8). Transforming growth factor demonstrates both inflammatory and anti-inflammatory effects. It may be at least partially responsible for tissue fibrosis associated with many diseases. It demonstrates immunosuppressive effects on T cells, B cells, and natural killer cells.

7. b Examples of Type II hypersensitivity include transfusion reactions, hemolytic disease of the newborn, autoimmune hemolytic anemia, Goodpasture's syndrome, and myasthenia gravis. In this form of hypersensitivity, antibody is directed against cell surface antigens, against small molecules adsorbed to cells, or against cell surface receptors, rather than against cell constituents themselves. Examples of type

I hypersensitivity include anaphylaxis, hay fever (allergic rhinitis) and, in some cases, asthma. Type III hypersensitivity may be associated with infections, such as hepatitis B and bacterial endocarditis; cancers, in which a serum sickness–like syndrome may occur; and autoimmune disorders such as lupus erythematosus. This hypersensitivity also may follow drug or serum therapy. Examples of Type IV hypersensitivity (delayed hypersensitivity) include tuberculin reactions, contact hypersensitivity, and sarcoidosis.

8. c Autoimmunity is characterized by a misdirected immune response, in which the body's defenses become self-destructive. In immunodeficiency, the immune response is absent or depressed, resulting in increased susceptibility to infection. In Type II hypersensitivity, binding of antigen and antibody activates complement, ultimately disrupting cellular membranes. In Type IV hypersensitivity sensitized T cells release lymphokines, and these and other activated pathways contribute to tissue damage.

Chapter 2:
Allergy

1. a Hay fever reflects an immunoglobulin E (IgE)-mediated Type I hypersensitivity response to an environmental antigen (allergen) in a genetically susceptible individual. It's usually induced by wind-borne pollens: in spring by tree pollens (oak, elm, maple, alder, birch, cottonwood); in summer by grass pollens (sheep sorrel, English plantain); and in fall by weed pollens (ragweed). Occasionally, hay fever is induced by allergy to fungal spores.

2. c Hay fever usually is accompanied by pale, cyanotic, edematous nasal mucosa; red (rather than pale), edematous eyelids and conjunctivae; and excessive lacrimation. In both perennial and seasonal allergic rhinitis, dark circles may appear under the patient's eyes ("allergic shiners") because of venous congestion in the maxillary sinuses. Eustachian tube obstruction is more apt to occur in perennial allergic rhinitis, especially in children. Beet red nasal mucosa occurs in infectious rhinitis (the common cold).

3. b Topical intranasal steroids combat local inflammation with minimal systemic adverse effects. The most commonly used drugs are flunisolide and beclomethasone. Newer antihistamines such as terfenadine and astemizole produce fewer adverse effects and are much less likely to cause sedation, but may induce ventricular arrhythmias, especially in patients with a prolonged QT interval or patients taking medications that prolong the QT interval, and especially with a high dose (overdose). Cromolyn sodium may help prevent allergic rhinitis but takes up to 4 weeks to produce desired effects. Desensitization with injections of extracted allergens controls all symptoms, but these are administered preseasonally, coseasonally, or perennially, with seasonal allergies requiring particularly close dosage regulation to prevent adverse reactions.

4. d Usually, the lesions of atopic dermatitis are located in areas of flexion and extension, such as the neck, antecubital fossa, and popliteal folds, and behind the ears. The eyelids and lips, genitalia, and mucous membranes are locations for angioedematous wheals. The chest and abdomen and palmar surface of the hands and soles of the feet are not primary locations for atopic dermatitis.

5. c Because dry skin aggravates itching, frequent application of nonirritating topical lubricants is important, especially after bathing or showering. Drying agents, such as calamine lotion, would further aggravate this problem. Topical corticosteroids help reduce inflammation in active dermatitis. Oral (systemic) antihistamines are commonly used to help control itching and reduce involuntary scratching during sleep.

6. d At the first sign of a hemolytic reaction (recipient immunoglobulin G [IgG] or IgM antibodies attach to donor red blood cells, resulting in widespread intravascular agglutination), immediately stop the transfusion (although some authorities recommend slowing the transfusion if the reaction is thought to be other than hemolytic). Keep the vein open with 0.9% sodium chloride solution until further determinations can be made. Administer antihistamines for allergic reactions (transfused soluble antigens react with surface IgE molecules on mast cells and basophils, releasing allergic mediators). Administer an antipyretic for a febrile nonhemolytic reaction (cytotoxic or agglutinated antibodies in the recipient's plasma attack antigens on transfused lympho-cytes, granulocytes, or plasma cells).

7. d Confirming a hemolytic transfusion reaction requires proof of blood incompatibility and evidence of hemolysis, such as hemoglobinuria, anti-A or anti-B antibodies in the serum (not the urine), and elevated bilirubin levels. If the patient requires mannitol or furosemide to maintain urinary function, hourly output and specific gravity levels measurements, and periodic measurements of creatinine clearance also will be required.

8. a Anaphylaxis requires immediate injection of epineph-rine 1:1,000 aqueous solution, 0.1 to 0.5 ml (S.C. or I.M. if the patient is conscious, I.V. if the patient is unconscious), re-peated every 5 to 20 minutes as needed. Aminophylline may be used for bronchospasm, and vasopressors such as nor-epinephrine and dopamine to stabilize blood pressure. Later, corticosteroids and diphenhydramine may be added for long-term management.

9. b Wheezing is the characteristic breath sound in asthma but is not a reliable indicator of severity. The intensity of breath sounds is typically reduced, with a prolonged phase of forced expiration. Wheezing may be accompanied by coarse gurgling sounds, but fine crackles are not heard un-less associated with a complication. Crackles in the bases of the lungs are heard with atelectasis. Laryngeal stridor is characteristic of laryngotracheal bronchitis (croup).

10. c Impaired consciousness (with symptoms of confusion and lethargy) is an ominous sign of respiratory failure in the patient with asthma. Partial pressure of carbon dioxide in-creases above 40 mm Hg; partial pressure of oxygen falls be-low 60 mm Hg; pH falls, demonstrating increasing respiratory acidosis; forced expiratory volume is decreased below 25%; and cyanosis may occur. Airway obstruction may be no worse, but the patient experiences fatigue and respiratory ef-fort decreases. In severe asthma, the patient has continuous symptoms and marked distress, but is still coping, despite the fact that bronchodilator therapy no longer fully reverses his airway obstruction. In status asthmaticus, asthma is persistent and intractable, and the patient is at high risk for respiratory failure without prompt treatment.

1. a Rheumatoid arthritis (RA) usually develops insidiously and initially produces nonspecific symptoms such as fatigue, malaise, anorexia, persistent low-grade fever, weight loss, lymphadenopathy, and vague articular symptoms. Later, more specific localized articular symptoms develop, frequently in the finger joints. These symptoms usually occur bilaterally and symmetrically and include stiffening of the affected joints after inactivity (particularly in the morning), marked joint edema and congestion, and joint tenderness and pain (upon movement at first, but eventually also at rest).

2. b Articular symptoms in RA may extend to the wrists, elbows, knees, and ankles. Hip and knee joints are frequently affected in osteoarthritis. Shoulders, hips, knees, and ankles, as well as costovertebral and sternomanubrial joints may be affected in ankylosing spondylitis.

3. b Volar subluxation and stretching of the tendons may pull the fingers to the ulnar side ("ulnar drift"). Rheumatoid nodules are extra-articular findings – subcutaneous, round or oval nontender masses – usually over bony prominences such as the elbows. Heberden's and Bouchard's nodes are bony, cartilaginous enlargements that develop on distal and proximal interphalangeal joints in osteoarthritis.

4. d Salicylates, particularly aspirin, are the mainstay of RA therapy because they decrease inflammation and relieve joint pain. Other useful medications include nonsteroidal anti-inflammatory agents or NSAIDs (such as indomethacin, fenoprofen, and ibuprofen), antimalarials (hydroxychloroquine), gold salts, penicillamine, and corticosteroids (prednisone). Immunosuppressives (cyclophosphamide, methotrexate, and azathioprine) are also therapeutic and are being used more commonly in early disease.

5. d Antimalarials are contraindicated in the treatment of psoriatic arthritis because these drugs can provoke exfoliative dermatitis. Treatment includes aspirin, NSAIDs, systemic corticosteroids, topical steroids, gold salts, and immunosuppressives, particularly methotrexate.

6. a Anti-inflammatory analgesics such as aspirin and indomethacin help to control pain and inflammation in ankylosing spondylitis, although no treatment reliably stops progression of the disease. Immunosuppressives, corticosteroids, and antimalarials are not used.

7. d Sjögren's syndrome, the second most common autoimmune rheumatic disorder after RA, is characterized by diminished lacrimal and salivary gland secretion. Urethritis, arthritis, and conjunctivitis characterize Reiter's syndrome. Nail changes, including pitting, transverse ridging, onycholysis, keratosis, yellowing, and destruction occur in psoriatic arthritis. Iridocyclitis may occur in juvenile RA.

8. b The classic butterfly rash across the nose and cheeks occurs in fewer than 50% of patients with systemic lupus erythematosus (SLE). However, this facial erythema remains the classic lesion associated with SLE. Polyarthralgia is very common, with 90% of SLE patients developing joint involvement similar to that of RA. Vasculitis can develop, possibly leading to infarctive lesions, necrotic ulcers, or digital gangrene. Raynaud's phenomenon appears in about 20% of patients.

9. c Urine studies in SLE patients, especially those with renal involvement, show excessive cellular casts and sediment in their urine and profuse proteinuria (>0.5 g/dl). Urine studies also may show some red blood cells and white blood cells; however hematuria indicates bleeding within the GU tract, which may result from infection, inflammation, obstruction, or trauma. Elevated porphyrins appear in congenital porphyrias (inherited enzyme deficiencies) or acquired porphyrias (as occur in hemolytic anemias and hepatic disease). Chronic bilateral pyelonephritis, acute or chronic glomerulonephritis, and polycystic kidney disease may depress urine creatinine levels.

10. d Cytotoxic drugs (azathioprine, methotrexate) may delay or prevent deteriorating renal status. Antihypertensive drugs (such as fosinopril, an angiotensin-converting enzyme inhibitor) and altered diet (low-protein, high-calorie, and sodium- and potassium-restricted, with added vitamin supplements) may also be warranted in renal disease. In diffuse proliferative glomerulonephritis, a major SLE complication, treatment is large doses of steroids (prednisone).

Chapter 4:
Immuno-
deficiency

1. d In X-linked infantile hypogammaglobulinemia, a mutation in the B-cell protein tyrosine kinase causes B cells to fail to mature and secrete immunoglobulins. B cells and B-cell precursors may be present in the bone marrow and peripheral blood. B cells do not die prematurely, but are unable to carry out their function because of immaturity. T cells are intact.

2. a Immune globulin is composed primarily of immunoglobulin G (IgG); thus the patient may also need fresh frozen plasma infusions to provide IgA and IgM. Unfortunately, mucosal secretory IgA cannot be replaced, resulting in frequent crippling pulmonary illnesses.

3. d To overcome problems associated with antibody testing, direct testing is performed to detect human immunodeficiency virus (HIV). Direct tests include antigen testing (p24 antigen), HIV cultures, nucleic probes of peripheral blood lymphocytes, and the polymerase chain reaction. Antibody tests such as the enzyme-linked immunosorbent assay (ELISA) are used for initial screening, with a positive ELISA repeated, then followed by an alternate method, usually the Western blot or immunofluorescence assay. Antibody tests may be unreliable because of the variable amount of time the body requires to produce a detectable level of antibodies. Thus, a negative ELISA or other antibody test does not necessarily indicate that HIV infection has not occurred.

4. c After a high-risk exposure and innoculation, the infected person usually experiences a mononucleosis-like syndrome, which may be attributed to flu or other virus. The infection then becomes latent, with the only sign being laboratory evidence of seroconversion. When symptoms appear after this latent period, they take many forms, including persistent, generalized lymphadenopathy; nonspecific symptoms; neurologic symptoms resulting from HIV encephalopathy; or an opportunistic infection (such as candidiasis) or malignancy.

5. c Zidovudine is effective in slowing the progression of HIV infection, decreasing opportunistic infections, and prolonging survival. Didanosine may be recommended for patients who cannot tolerate, or who no longer respond to, zidovudine therapy. Zalcitabine is used in combination with zidovudine in advanced acquired immunodeficiency syndrome (AIDS) to enhance the return of CD4$^+$ T-lymphocyte levels. Pentamidine may be used I.V. or in aerosol form to treat *Pneumocystis carinii* pneumonia.

6. b Neurologic dysfunction (AIDS dementia complex, HIV encephalopathy, and peripheral neuropathies) occurs because of direct destruction of neuroglial cells by HIV infection. Direct destruction of CD4$^+$ cells and other immune cells, and, indirectly, secondary effects of CD4$^+$ T-lymphocyte dysfunction and resultant immunosuppression lead to immunodeficiency (opportunistic infections and unusual cancers) and to autoimmunity (lymphoid interstitial pneumonitis, hypergammaglobulinemia, and production of autoimmune antibodies).

7. a The cause of chronic fatigue and immune dysfunction syndrome is unknown, but researchers suspect it may be found in human herpesvirus-6 or in other herpesviruses, enteroviruses, or retroviruses. Rising levels of antibodies to the Epstein-Barr virus (EBV), once thought to implicate EBV infection as the cause of chronic fatigue and immune dysfunction syndrome, are now considered a result of this disease. Chronic fatigue and immune dysfunction syndrome may be associated with a reaction to a viral illness (rather than a bacterial one) that is complicated by a dysfunctional immune response. An inherited defect in the cell-mediated (T-cell) immune system may cause chronic mucocutaneous candidiasis.

8. c *Pneumocystis carinii* pneumonia usually strikes a severely immunodeficient infant with severe combined immunodeficiency disease in the first few weeks of life. Within the first few months of life, this infant commonly develops recurrent pulmonary infections, often caused by *Pseudo-monas* or cytomegalovirus; persistent oral candidiasis, sometimes with esophageal erosions; and common viral infections (such as chickenpox) that are often fatal. Because of complete immunodeficiency (both T-cell and B-cell immunity are absent or deficient), this infant also would be at risk for mycobacterial and fungal infections, including histoplasmosis.

9. d C2 and C4 complement deficiencies are associated with collagen vascular disease, such as lupus erythematosus, and chronic renal failure. C2 and C3 deficiencies and C5 familial dysfunction increase susceptibility to bacterial infections. C5 dysfunction, a familial defect in infants, causes failure to thrive, diarrhea, and seborrheic dermatitis. C1 esterase inhibitor deficiency, also known as hereditary angioedema, may cause periodic swelling in the face, hands, abdomen, or throat, with potential fatal laryngeal edema.

10. b Life-threatening hypocalcemia must be treated immediately in DiGeorge's syndrome. It's unusually resistant and requires aggressive therapy, often with rapid I.V. infusion of a 10% calcium gluconate solution, along with vitamin D and, sometimes, also with parathyroid hormone. After hypocalcemia is under control, fetal thymic transplant may restore normal cell-mediated immunity. Cardiac anomalies require surgical repair where possible. Facial anomalies are repaired cosmetically as necessary if the patient survives infancy.

Appendices and Index

Organ-Specific Autoimmune Disorders

DISORDER	IMMUNOLOGIC FEATURES AND TEST FINDINGS	SIGNS AND SYMPTOMS	INTERVENTIONS
Cardiac disorders			
Acute rheumatic fever	• Follows group A streptococcal pharyngitis, which may have occurred a few days to 6 weeks earlier • Genetic predisposition • Formation of antibodies to streptococcal cellular and extracellular antigens • Presence of cross-reactive antibodies that bind to various host tissues • Presence of lymphocytes that are cytotoxic to cardiac tissue • Elevated white blood cell (WBC) count, erythrocyte sedimentation rate (ESR), and C-reactive protein level • Positive group A streptococcal throat culture • Prolonged PR interval on electrocardiogram (ECG) in 20% of patients • Increased antistreptolysin O or other streptococcal antibody • Cardiac catheterization to evaluate left ventricular function and valvular damage, both present in severe cardiac dysfunction • Echocardiography to evaluate valvular damage, chamber size, and ventricular function	• Episode of pharyngitis about 2 to 3 weeks before onset of acute rheumatic symptoms • Arthritis, also known as migratory joint pain or polyarthritis (pain, redness, swelling, and warmth of affected joints) • Cardiac inflammation leading to heart failure, dyspnea, and mitral and aortic murmurs • Purposeless movements of voluntary muscles, aggravated by stress and alleviated during sleep or rest (Sydenham's chorea) • Circular erythematous rash, commonly on trunk and proximal parts of limbs • Fever over 100.4° F (38° C), periumbilical pain • Subcutaneous nodules, firm, moveable, nontender nodules 3 mm to 2 cm in diameter near tendons or bony prominences	• Antibiotics (usually penicillin or erythromycin) initiated during acute phase • Bed rest for 5 weeks during acute phase with carditis • Symptomatic treatment, such as salicylates for arthritic symptoms, initiated during acute phase • Possibly, diuretics, valvular surgery, and commissurotomy

DISORDER	IMMUNOLOGIC FEATURES AND TEST FINDINGS	SIGNS AND SYMPTOMS	INTERVENTIONS
Cardiac disorders *(continued)*			
Postcardiac injury syndrome (Dressler's syndrome, postmyocardial infarction syndrome, postpericardiotomy syndrome)	• Elevated levels of antibodies to viral agents • Circulating antibodies to cardiac tissue • Circulating lymphocytes sensitized to mitochondrial extracts of cardiac tissue • Increased WBC count and ESR, positive test for circulating anticardiac antibodies (if available) • ECG with elevated ST segments in standard limb leads without significant QRS morphology changes • Supportive diagnosis from echocardiogram that reveals echo-free space between ventricular wall and pericardium • Slightly elevated cardiac enzyme levels with associated myocarditis	• Fever after first week following surgery, trauma, or myocardial infarction • Pericarditis (pericardial friction rub, chest pain) pleuritic-type pain (increases with deep inspiration and decreases when patient sits up, leans forward and, therefore, pulls heart away from diaphragmatic pleurae of lungs) • Pleural effusion • Pericardial effusion • Pericardial friction rub • Cardiac tamponade • Large pericardial effusion, neck vein distention, pulsus paradoxus, dyspnea, and shock	• Aspirin for pain or indomethacin to decrease inflammation • Corticosteroids in severe cases • Pericardiocentesis if cardiac tamponade develops • Bed rest as long as fever and pain persist
Dermatologic disorders			
Bullous pemphigoid	• Separation of epidermis from dermis at lamina lucida • Benign, chronic, self-limiting course • Immunoglobulin and complement deposits on skin's basement membrane • Serum anti-skin basement membrane antibody (present in 80% of patients) • Passive in vivo transfer of the disease with human pemphigoid antibody • Neutrophil and eosinophil chemotactic factors in blister fluid	• Commonly affects elderly patients • Tense, subepidermal, difficult-to-rupture bullae in flexor areas (inguinal, axillae, sides of neck) • Severe pruritus • May be accompanied by annular, dusky-red edematous lesions with or without peripheral vesicles • Rapidly healing oral lesions	• Corticosteroid therapy, sometimes combined with azathioprine • Good skin hygiene

(continued)

DISORDER	IMMUNOLOGIC FEATURES AND TEST FINDINGS	SIGNS AND SYMPTOMS	INTERVENTIONS
Dermatologic disorders *(continued)*			
Pemphigus vulgaris	• Immunoglobin and complement deposits in squamous intracellular spaces • May resemble burn injury • If untreated, will progress to death by fluid and electrolyte loss and sepsis • Serum antibody directed against intercellular substance of stratified squamous epithelium • Pemphigus immunoglobulin G (IgG) promoting epidermal cell detachment in vitro and in vivo • Increased incidence of human leukocyte antigen known as HLA-Dw4	• Thin, flaccid bullae within the epidermis (intraepidermal blister), especially on trunk and scalp, but with no characteristic distribution • Ruptured bullae extend in size • Skin easily denuded by shearing force • Oral and nasal mucosal involvement; extensive oral erosion • Commonly affects middle-aged or elderly patients • Pruritus and pain with lesions	• Administration of immunosuppressants, such as azathioprine, methotrexate, or cyclophosphamide and I.M. gold alone or with corticosteroids, until remission occurs • Plasmapheresis combined with immunosuppressants • Fluid, electrolyte, and nutritional support • Monitoring for complications of therapy: GI bleeding, osteoporosis, and diabetes
Endocrine disorders			
Addison's disease (idiopathic adrenocortical insufficiency)	• Autoantibodies to adrenal microsomes • Lymphocytic and monocytic infiltration of adrenal glands • Other autoimmune autoantibodies (to thyroid, parathyroid, or gonadal tissue) • Low serum and urine cortisol levels	• Postural hypotension, weight loss, anorexia, weakness, and cutaneous and mucosal pigmentation • Other autoimmune diseases: diabetes mellitus, ovarian failure, and Hashimoto's thyroiditis • Possible additional disorders: pernicious anemia, vitiligo, alopecia, nontropical sprue, and myasthenia gravis	• Replacement of glucocorticoids and mineralocorticoids • Symptomatic and supportive care as needed

DISORDER	IMMUNOLOGIC FEATURES AND TEST FINDINGS	SIGNS AND SYMPTOMS	INTERVENTIONS
Endocrine disorders *(continued)*			
Chronic thyroiditis (Hashimoto's thyroiditis)	• Thyroid function tests elevated, depressed, or normal • Autoantibodies to thyroglobulin or thyroid microsomes or both • Decreased thyroid hormone levels and radioactive iodine uptake in later stages; elevated serum thyroid-stimulating hormone and serum cholesterol levels • Self-limited or responsive to thyroid hormone treatment	• Diffusely enlarged thyroid, producing goiter usually firm to hard, only rarely tender, and smooth or scalloped without distinct nodules • Diminished thyroid function in later stages, suggesting failure of epithelial cell regeneration • Dry skin; coarse, brittle hair; possible myxedema • Low basal metabolic rate	• Administration of thyroid hormone (synthetic thyroxine) • Corticosteroids or immunosuppressants to relieve inflammation • Supportive and symptomatic care • Surgery or radioactive iodine usually not recommended
Diabetes mellitus (type I)	• Circulating antibodies against islet cells • Infiltration of beta cells by activated T lymphocytes, primarily T-suppressor cells but also T-helper cells and natural killer cells • Abnormal deposits of IgG and complement • Both humoral and cell-mediated autoimmune phenomena, the latter being more important • Expression of selective aberrant HLA-DR • Possible link to viral infection	• Abrupt onset of polyuria, polydipsia, polyphagia, weight loss, and fatigue	• Insulin • Dietary modifications • Exercise • Supportive and symptomatic care
Graves' disease	• Autoantibodies directed to thyroid cell surface receptors for thyrotropin or thyroid-stimulating hormone (TSH) • Thyrotropin receptor antibodies that either mimic the stimulatory action of TSH or block TSH binding • Autoantibodies to thyroglobulin or thyroid microsomes, identified by a combination of hemagglutination and immunofluorescence tests • Elevated serum levels of thyroxine and triiodothyronine	• Diffuse goiter • Restlessness, heat intolerance, weight loss, and palpitations • Tachycardia, widened pulse pressure, and elevated systolic pressure • Fine tremor of hands and proximal muscle weakness • Exophthalmos • Dermopathy characterized by raised, thickened skin (usually over dorsum of legs or feet) that has	• Thyroidectomy, administration of radioactive iodine, or antithyroid drugs and adjunctive use of iodine or adrenergic blocking agents • Treatment with immunosuppressants rarely necessary (Restoration of normal hormone balance appears to decrease inflammation and arrest disease.) *(continued)*

DISORDER	IMMUNOLOGIC FEATURES AND TEST FINDINGS	SIGNS AND SYMPTOMS	INTERVENTIONS
Endocrine disorders *(continued)*			
Graves' disease *(continued)*	• Increased uptake of radioactive iodine by thyroid	a peau d'orange appearance and may be pruritic and hyperpigmented	
GI disorders			
Chronic active hepatitis	• Autoantibodies to liver membrane, smooth muscle, and nuclear antigens • Genetic association with HLA-B8 and HLA-Dw3 • Defect in nonspecific immunoregulation associated with polyclonal hypergammaglobulinemia • Elevated serum bilirubin and aminotransferase levels • Normal or slightly elevated alkaline phosphatase levels • Low serum albumin level and prolonged prothrombin time • Elevated serum IgG, anti-DNA, and antinuclear antibodies	• Usually insidious onset over several weeks to months • Chronic hepatic inflammation continuing without improvement for longer than 6 months • Fatigue • Persistent or recurrent jaundice • Malaise for several months before jaundice appears • Anorexia • Recurrent, worsening symptoms suggesting acute hepatitis • Complications of cirrhosis (ascites, bleeding esophageal varices, encephalopathy, coagulopathy, hypersplenism)	• Supportive care with adequate rest; then activity as tolerated when remission occurs • Corticosteroids in moderate or low doses, sometimes combined with azathioprine • Continuing drug therapy for at least 6 to 12 months, possibly for life if relapse occurs on withdrawal • High-dose corticosteroid therapy for patients unresponsive to other therapy
Inflammatory bowel disease (Crohn's disease, ulcerative colitis)	• Increased numbers of lymphocytes, plasma cells, and monocytes in the mucosa and, in Crohn's disease, the submucosa • Granulomatous response in intestinal lesions and regional lymph nodes in Crohn's disease • Presence of circulating antibodies to cytoplasmic lipopolysaccharides of epithelial cells in colon • Circulating lymphocytotoxic antibodies • Low serum protein levels, serum electrolyte abnormalities • Elevated ESR	• Mild to severe diarrhea; dehydration and electrolyte imbalances in severe diarrhea • Bloody stools • Lower abdominal pain • Fever • Bowel perforation (more common in ulcerative colitis) • Fistula formation between portions of the bowel itself or communicating with skin (perianal), vagina, or bladder (more common in Crohn's disease)	• Fluid and blood replacement as needed • Corticosteroids and sulfasalazine in colitis; possibly given with azathioprine to allow reduced corticosteroid dosages • Metronidazole in Crohn's disease • Surgical resection of affected area (Total colectomy to cure ulcerative colitis; Crohn's disease may recur in another segment after resection.)

DISORDER	IMMUNOLOGIC FEATURES AND TEST FINDINGS	SIGNS AND SYMPTOMS	INTERVENTIONS
GI disorders *(continued)*			
Inflammatory bowel disease (Crohn's disease, ulcerative colitis) *(continued)*		• Malabsorption syndrome with malnutrition when small bowel is involved • Oral ulcers in Crohn's disease • Extraintestinal disease symptoms; lesions of eyes, joints, skin, liver, and biliary tracts • Colon cancer (after 10 or more years of colitis) • Anemia resulting from intestinal blood loss and poor nutrient absorption	• Nutritional support, possibly oral or total parenteral nutrition
Primary biliary cirrhosis	• Presence of mitochondrial antibodies • Diminished suppressor cell function • Increased serum immunoglobulin M (IgM) levels • Inability to convert from IgM to IgG antibody synthesis • Complement-activating serum factor, possibly immune complexes • Granulomatous infiltrates in intrahepatic biliary tree • Markedly elevated serum alkaline phosphate levels • Normal or slightly elevated serum transaminase levels • Elevated serum copper levels	• Pruritus • Hyperlipidemia (especially hypercholesterolemia) with resulting xanthomas (yellowish lipid plaques in subcutaneous tissues) in periorbital areas, skin folds, and trauma sites • Steatorrhea and fat-soluble vitamin malabsorption after cholestasis develops, with resulting intestinal bile salt deficiency • Jaundice, dark urine, light stools • Anergy • Signs of portal hypertension and liver insufficiency • Metabolic bone disease with vertebral compression fractures	• Antihistamines, topical lotions, or cholestyramine for pruritus • Penicillamine for copper-chelating and anti-inflammatory effects • Substitution of dietary medium-chain triglycerides for long-chain triglycerides to reduce steatorrhea • Parenteral administration of fat-soluble vitamins D, A, and K • Plasmapheresis

(continued)

DISORDER	IMMUNOLOGIC FEATURES AND TEST FINDINGS	SIGNS AND SYMPTOMS	INTERVENTIONS
Hematologic disorders			
Autoimmune neutropenia	• Antineutrophil antibodies noted by agglutination or by immunofluorescence tests • Severe neutropenia (less than 500/mm³) • Occurs with transfusion reactions or after viral infection; associated with other autoimmune diseases, such as systemic lupus erythematosus, and with lymphoreticular malignancies, such as Hodgkin's disease	• Infections • Splenomegaly • Abdominal pain • Fatigue • Circulating large granular lymphocytes with normal to increased count • Normal monocyte, erythrocyte, and platelet counts • Normal or increased marrow cellularity; decreased mature neutrophil count	• Infection prevention strategies • High-dose I.V. immune globulin • Antithymocyte globulin (investigational) • Plasmapheresis (investigational) • Glucocorticoid therapy
Autoimmune thrombocytopenic purpura	• Abnormal bleeding time • Antiplatelet antibodies on platelets and in serum • Decreased platelet survival time • Depressed platelet count (acute, less than 30,000/mm³; chronic, 30,000 to 100,000/mm³) • Therapeutic response to prednisone and splenectomy	• Left-sided abdominal pain accompanying splenomegaly • Usually acute onset • With acute onset, fever • Petechiae, ecchymoses, epistaxis, and gingival, GI, or genitourinary bleeding • Possible cerebral hemorrhage • Acute systemic illness with fever (in thrombocytopenia associated with another disease) • Splenomegaly likely • Moderate anemia resulting from blood loss and iron deficiency	• I.V. gamma globulin in cases of decreased IgG levels • Cryoprecipitate if traditional therapies fail • Avoid I.M. injections in low platelet counts. • Avoidance of drugs associated with platelet or coagulation abnormalities • Monitoring of vascular volume and oxygenation if severe bleeding occurs • Withdrawal of offending drug in suspected drug-induced thrombocytopenia • In children, treatment often not needed; corticosteroids in severe thrombocytopenia and bleeding • Splenectomy in adults; immunosuppressants if splenectomy fails • If life-threatening bleeding occurs, high-dose I.V. immune globulin and platelet concentrates

DISORDER	IMMUNOLOGIC FEATURES AND TEST FINDINGS	SIGNS AND SYMPTOMS	INTERVENTIONS
Hematologic disorders *(continued)*			
Pernicious anemia	• Evidence of both humoral and cell-mediated immunity to gastric mucosal antigens • High incidence of antiparietal cell antibodies • Autoantibodies to gastric parietal cells and vitamin B_{12} binding site of intrinsic factor • Parietal cell cytotoxicity	• Pallor, fatigue, progressive muscle weakness • Anorexia, weight loss • Neurologic involvement, including peripheral neuropathies, damage to pyramidal tract and posterior column neurons, and disturbances in higher cortical function • Macrocytic anemia and hypersegmentation of nuclei of neutrophil granulocytes, detected on peripheral blood smear • Megaloblastosis on examination of bone marrow aspirate • Serum B_{12} level below 120 pg/ml (normally 200 to 1,500 pg/ml)	• Regular I.M. injections of vitamin B_{12} • Corticosteroid or immunosuppressant therapy (experimental)
Warm antibody autoimmune hemolytic anemia	• Most common form of autoimmune hemolytic anemia • Shortened red blood cell (RBC) survival • Presence of spherocytes on peripheral smear • About half of cases are related to malignancy • Drugs linked to occurrence of syndrome (including methyldopa or levodopa)	• Jaundice with hyperbilirubinemia (primarily unconjugated) • Positive urinary bilinogen • Low serum haptoglobin levels • Other clinical signs and symptoms of anemia—for example, angina and dyspnea • Reticulocyte count usually elevated (although possibly reduced after a prolonged course of the disease)	• Possible plasmapheresis or plasma exchange, but results are inconclusive • Adminstration of vinblastine-loaded, IgG-sensitized platelets causing splenic injury • Treatment of underlying disease process • High-dose corticosteroid therapy • Splenectomy if corticosteroid therapy fails *(continued)*

DISORDER	IMMUNOLOGIC FEATURES AND TEST FINDINGS	SIGNS AND SYMPTOMS	INTERVENTIONS
Hematologic disorders *(continued)*			
Warm antibody autoimmune hemolytic anemia *(continued)*	• Occurs in children after acute infection or immunization • Commonly takes chronic course featuring relapses and remissions • Positive direct antiglobulin (Coombs') test • Increased unconjugated serum bilirubin levels • Possibly associated with lymphoreticular malignancy or autoimmune disease	• Thromboembolic episodes (such as thrombophlebitis, pulmonary emboli, and splenic infarcts) common causes of morbidity • Splenomegaly • Anemia and signs of hemolysis • Leukocytosis and thrombocytosis • Occurs more frequently in women than in men	• Immunosuppressants if corticosteroids and splenectomy fail • Blood transfusion, if required, to prevent serious complication of anemia (Transfusion is avoided, if possible, because transfused blood is rapidly destroyed.)
Cold antibody autoimmune hemolytic anemia	• Two types: cold agglutin antibodies and paroxysmal cold hemoglobinuria (Donath-Landsteiner test) • Shortened RBC survival • Associated with lymphoreticular malignancies (half of cases) • Commonly associated with certain infections (infectious mononucleosis, mycoplasmal pneumonia, Epstein-Barr virus)	• In disorder associated with complement activation, severe and massive hemolysis with body cooling • Massive hemolysis likely to present as anemia, hyperbilirubinemia, shock, acrocyanosis, and hemoglobinuria • Self-limiting hemolysis symptoms (most prominent after body cooling and resolving with rewarming) • Thromboembolic episodes (such as thrombophlebitis, pulmonary emboli, and splenic infarcts) common causes of morbidity	• Patient warmth maintained by wrapping extremities or using warming blankets as needed • Limits imposed on operating room time or procedures requiring massive blood transfusions • Blood product administration limited, if possible • All RBCs administered through a blood warmer • In severe cases, washed RBCs given to reduce risk of reactions • Chlorambucil or cyclophosphamide useful in some cases • Glucocorticoids in severe cases only • Plasma exchange with albumin-containing saline solution for temporary relief of hemolytic symptoms

DISORDER	IMMUNOLOGIC FEATURES AND TEST FINDINGS	SIGNS AND SYMPTOMS	INTERVENTIONS
Neurologic disorders			
Multiple sclerosis	• Inflammatory demyelination of central nervous system (CNS) white matter • Increased IgG level in cerebrospinal fluid (CSF), with oligoclonal bands • Elevated antiviral antibody levels in serum and CSF • Elevated levels of total protein (during acute phase) and myelin basic protein in CSF • Multiple sclerosis plaques detected by magnetic resonance imaging	• Motor weakness, paresthesia • Impaired visual acuity, diplopia • Ataxia, urinary bladder dysfunction, impotence, spasticity • Acute exacerbations of signs and symptoms that persist for days to weeks with gradual recovery (more slowly in chronic, progressive disease) • Mild to moderate dementia (late)	• Symptomatic and supportive care • Corticosteroids, immunosuppressants, and plasmapheresis to shorten periods of exacerbation or to arrest disease progress • Interferon alfa and interferon beta for remitting and relapsing multiple sclerosis
Myasthenia gravis	• Commonly associated with thymoma or thymic hyperplasia • Pathogenic autoantibodies directed against acetylcholine-receptor protein in serum • Often associated with other autoimmune diseases, such as rheumatoid arthritis or systemic lupus erythematosis • Positive Tensilon test results for diagnostic confirmation	• Muscles often weak or normal at rest, becoming increasingly weaker with repetitive use • Skeletal muscle weakness usually proximal, causing difficulty in climbing stairs, rising from chairs, combing hair, even holding up head • Weakness of extraocular muscles, manifested as diplopia or ptosis—usually unilateral • Pharyngeal and facial muscle weakness resulting in dysphagia, dysarthria, and difficulty chewing	• Anticholinesterase drugs • Thymectomy • Corticosteroids and also immunosuppressants for patients unresponsive to anticholinesterase drugs or thymectomy or as an adjunct to routine therapy • Plasmapheresis

Chief Complaints in Immune Disorders

Several important signs and symptoms—fever, fatigue, weight loss, lymphadenopathy, joint pain, and rash—occur in patients with immune disorders. (Many of these also occur in patients with infectious disorders.) By fully investigating these complaints, you can form a diagnostic impression of your patient's problem and guide your subsequent care.

Fever

A body temperature above 98.6° F (37° C), fever commonly arises from disorders in virtually every body system. It has little diagnostic value by itself. Cytokines produced by macrophages, especially interleukin-1, alter the thermoregulatory center and represent the ultimate cause of most fevers.

Fever commonly occurs in hypersensitivity reactions, acquired immunodeficiency syndrome (AIDS), autoimmune hemolytic anemia, and autoimmune connective tissue diseases, such as rheumatoid arthritis, systemic lupus erythematosus, and progressive systemic sclerosis.

Fever can be classified as low (an oral reading of 99° to 100.4° F, or 37.2° to 38° C), moderate (100.5 to 104° F, or 38.1° to 40° C), or high (above 104° F). Fever above 105° F (40.6° C) constitutes a medical emergency. Fever above 106° F (41.1° C) causes unconsciousness and, if prolonged, brain damage. You should report any fever above 101° F (38.3°C) to the doctor.

If the patient's fever approaches 105° F (40.6° C), take his other vital signs and assess his level of consciousness. Administer antipyretic drugs and begin the following rapid cooling measures: Apply ice packs to the axillae and groin, give tepid sponge baths, and apply a hypothermia blanket. To prevent a rebound hypothermic response, constantly monitor the patient's rectal temperature.

If the patient's fever is low to moderate, proceed with the health history and physical examination according to the guidelines below.

History of the sign
To further explore your patient's fever, consider asking him the following questions:
• How long have you had the fever?
• What was your highest temperature?
• Did the fever begin suddenly or gradually?
• Did it rise steadily or rise, fall, and then rise again?
• Have you been exposed to high environmental temperatures for a prolonged period? If so, how much fluid did you drink?
• Have you recently been exposed to someone with the flu or any other infection?
• In your occupation or leisure activities, do you work with soil?
• Do you have any pets, or have you been exposed to wild animals?
• Have you traveled recently?

Associated findings
Ask the patient if he has experienced any of the following signs or symptoms:
• pain
• changes in level of consciousness (LOC)
• chills, fatigue, or sore throat
• swollen glands
• persistent cough
• morning stiffness
• nocturnal diaphoresis
• skin lesions or open areas that appear inflamed
• pruritus
• diarrhea, anorexia, or weight loss
• oliguria, burning upon urination, or any other urinary changes.

Previous conditions and treatments
Consult with the patient, family members, or members of the health care team to determine if the patient has ever had any of the following conditions, treatments, or risk factors:
• surgery or diagnostic testing
• blood transfusion
• bone marrow transplant

• immunizations
• infection
• burns or other traumatic injury
• endocrine dysfunction
• malignant hypertension
• autoimmune disorder
• immunosuppressive treatment, such as chemotherapy or radiation therapy
• immunosuppressive disorder, such as AIDS
• physical or emotional stress
• allergy
• asthma.

Drug history
Various drugs can cause a hypersensitivity reaction leading to fever. These include:
• penicillins
• procainamide
• sulfonamides.
   Toxic doses of the following drugs may also cause fever:
• salicylates
• amphetamines
• tricyclic antidepressants.
   Inhaled anesthetics and muscle relaxants can trigger malignant hyperthermia in genetically predisposed patients. Chemotherapeutic drugs may also cause fever.

Physical examination
Examine the patient according to the steps described below.
• Assess the patient's vital signs. Check especially for tachycardia and tachypnea.
• Assess LOC and mental status. Be alert for signs of restlessness, irritability, or seizure activity. Also note malaise, fatigue, or anxiety.
• Inspect skin color. Note if the patient's face appears flushed and whether diaphoresis or shivering is present.
• Inspect for signs of dehydration, such as a dry, furrowed tongue.
• Inspect lymph nodes for visible swelling or redness.
• Observe motor activity for possible muscle tremors and twitching.
   Let the health history findings guide the remainder of the physical examination.

Fatigue

Fatigue is commonly reported as tiredness, exhaustion, a lack of energy, or a strong desire to rest or sleep. It may be accompanied by weakness, which involves the muscles.
   Fatigue may represent a normal response to physical overexertion and sleep deprivation or a nonspecific symptom of psychological or physiologic disorders. It may be acute or chronic and commonly accompanies immune disorders.
   Fatigue commonly occurs in acquired immunodeficiency syndrome, systemic lupus erythematosus, rheumatoid arthritis, myasthenia gravis, pernicious anemia, autoimmune hemolytic anemia, Addison's disease, and insulin-dependent diabetes mellitus.
   If your patient complains of fatigue, take his health history and perform a physical examination according to the guidelines below.

History of the symptom
To explore your patient's complaint of fatigue, consider asking him the following questions:
• When did you first feel unusually tired?
• How long have you felt this way?
• How would you rate your fatigue on a scale of 1 (no fatigue) to 10 (extreme fatigue)?
• During what part of the day are you most tired?
• Is your fatigue related to activity?
• Does rest help?
• What makes you feel better? Worse?
• Has fatigue affected your daily activities? If so, how?
• Have you recently experienced unusual stress?
• Has your nutritional intake recently changed?

Associated findings
Ask the patient if he has experienced any of the following signs or symptoms:
• shortness of breath or other respiratory difficulty
• pain or unusual bleeding

- weakness or loss of consciousness
- nocturia
- insomnia
- nausea, vomiting, or diarrhea
- feelings of anxiety or depression
- recent weight changes
- persistent cough
- fever.

Previous conditions and treatments
Consult with the patient, family members, or members of the health care team to determine if the patient has ever had any of the following disorders, risk factors, or treatments:
- cancer
- heart or kidney disease
- chronic obstructive pulmonary disease
- anemia
- diabetes mellitus
- multiple sclerosis
- recent surgery
- rheumatic disease
- mental illness.

Drug history
Obtain a drug history and note past or current use of drugs that may cause fatigue, such as:
- antihypertensives, especially beta blockers
- sedatives
- corticosteroids
- amiodarone
- carbamazepine
- flecainide
- recombinant interferon alfa-2a or alfa-2b, interferon alfa-n3 (derived from human leukocytes), interferon gamma 1-b, or recombinant interleukin-2
- pentamidine isethionate for inhalation
- clomipramine
- dantrolene
- metoclopramide
- etretinate.

Physical examination
Observe the patient's general appearance for signs of depression or organic illness. Note whether he appears pale, unkempt, expressionless, tired, underweight, or otherwise unhealthy.

Assess his mental status, noting especially any of the following characteristics:
- agitation

- poor attention span
- confusion
- psychomotor impairment.

Depending on the history, you may need to assess a body system more closely or perform a thorough physical examination.

Weight loss

Weight loss may result from decreased food intake, increased metabolic requirements, impaired absorption of nutrients, loss of nutrients in urine or feces, or treatment of fluid retention. Nearly any serious illness can cause weight loss.

Weight loss is a major sign in patients with acquired immunodeficiency syndrome and commonly occurs in patients with Crohn's disease, insulin-dependent diabetes mellitus, hyperthyroidism, ulcerative colitis, Addison's disease, rheumatoid arthritis, progressive systemic sclerosis, and other connective tissue disorders, such as ankylosing spondylitis, polymyalgia, rheumatism, and polymyositis with dermatomyositis.

If your patient complains of weight loss, take his health history and perform a physical examination according to the guidelines below.

History of the sign
To further understand your patient's weight loss, consider asking him the following questions:
- When did you first notice you were losing weight?
- Has your weight loss stopped or are you still losing weight?
- How much weight have you lost?
- Over how long a period have you been losing weight?
- Was your weight loss intentional?
- Have your eating habits changed? Would you say that you are eating about the same amount, more than usual, or less than usual? If less than usual, do you know why?
- Have you recently felt anxious or depressed?
- Do you have any problems obtaining or preparing food? Chewing food?
- How do you feel about your weight loss?

Associated findings

Note whether the patient has experienced any of the following signs or symptoms:
• anorexia, diarrhea, or vomiting
• polyuria or excessive thirst
• steatorrhea
• dysphagia
• fever
• pain
• lymphadenopathy
• fatigue
• stomatitis.

Previous conditions and treatments

Consult with the patient, family members, or members of the health care team to determine if the patient has ever had any of the following conditions, treatments, or risk factors:
• cancer
• alcoholism or drug abuse
• diabetes mellitus or other endocrine diseases
• gastrointestinal disease
• recent surgery
• trauma
• psychosocial factors, such as poverty or social isolation
• human immunodeficiency virus infection, high-risk sexual activity, I.V. drug abuse, or blood transfusions between 1977 and 1988.

Drug history

Ask the patient about past or current use of the drugs listed below:
• diuretics
• appetite suppressants
• thyroid preparations
• laxatives
• chemotherapeutic drugs
• interferon gamma 1-b, recombinant interferon alfa-2a, or interleukin-2
• alprazolam
• guanadrel
• tolmetin
• bupropion.

Physical examination

Carefully check the patient's height, weight, and vital signs, including temperature, blood pressure, respiratory rate and depth, and pulse rate and rhythm. Assess his general appearance. Be sure to note any of the following findings:

• evidence of malnourishment or overly loose clothing
• signs of muscle wasting
• skin turgor and abnormal pigmentation, especially around the joints
• jaundice or pallor
• sparse and dry hair
• signs of infection or irritation on the roof of the mouth
• swelling in the neck or ankles.

Palpate the patient's liver for enlargement and tenderness. Let the health history guide the remainder of the physical examination.

Lymphadenopathy

Normally, lymph nodes are discrete, mobile, nontender, and nonpalpable, ranging in size from 0.5 to 2.5 cm. The presence of nodes larger than 3 cm indicates lymphadenopathy and is cause for concern. Lymph nodes may be tender and erythematous (suggesting a draining lesion), hard and fixed, and tender or nontender.

Enlargement of one or more lymph nodes may be generalized or localized. Generalized lymphadenopathy (involving three or more node groups) may stem from connective tissue disease, an endocrine disorder, a neoplastic disorder, or an inflammatory process, such as bacterial or viral infection. Localized lymphadenopathy (involving one or two node groups) commonly results from infection or trauma affecting the drained area.

Lymphadenopathy commonly occurs in acquired immunodeficiency syndrome and in other immunodeficiency disorders associated with opportunistic infections. It also occurs in rheumatoid arthritis, Sjögren's syndrome, systemic lupus erythematosus, serum sickness, and sarcoidosis.

If your patient reports swollen lymph nodes, take his health history and perform a physical examination according to the guidelines that follow.

History of the sign

To further explore your patient's swollen lymph nodes, consider asking the following questions:
• When did you first notice the swelling?

• Are the swollen areas painful?
• Have you recently had a cold, a virus, or any other health problems?

Associated findings
Note whether the patient has experienced any of the following signs or symptoms:
• fever
• pain
• fatigue
• weight loss
• night sweats
• purulent drainage.

Previous conditions and treatments
Consult with the patient, family members, or members of the health care team to determine if the patient has ever had any of the following disorders, risk factors, or treatments:
• valvular heart disease
• cancer
• trauma
• biopsy or surgery
• sexually transmitted disease or other infection, including human immunodeficiency virus infection
• high-risk sexual activity
• I.V. drug abuse
• blood transfusion between 1977 and 1988.

Drug history
Ask the patient about past and current use of the following drugs:
• phenytoin
• hydralazine
• allopurinol
• typhoid vaccine.

Physical examination
Assess the patient's height, weight, and vital signs, including temperature, blood pressure, respiratory rate and depth, and pulse rate and rhythm. Then examine him according to the steps that follow.

Inspection
• Note if the patient appears tired, cachectic, flushed, or in distress.
• Inspect his mouth and pharynx for redness, swelling, and exudation.
• Note needle tracks or wounds of any type.

Palpation
• Palpate all lymph nodes to determine the extent of lymphadenopathy and to detect any other areas of local enlargement.
• Use the pads of your index and middle fingers to move the skin over underlying tissues at the nodal area. Note the location and extent of enlarged lymph nodes.
• Record the size of enlarged nodes in centimeters, and note if they're fixed or mobile, tender or nontender, and pale or reddened. Is the node discrete or does the area feel matted?
• If you detect tender, hot nodes, check the area drained by them for signs of infection, such as erythema and swelling.

Let the patient's history and the lymph node assessment guide the remainder of the physical examination.

Joint pain

Any disorder involving inflammation or degeneration of joints or surrounding structures may cause pain. Joint pain may also stem from joint overuse or trauma. It may restrict range of motion and interfere with the ability to perform daily activities.

In certain disorders, pain may affect one joint (for example, bursitis, tendinitis, or injury); other disorders, such as rheumatoid arthritis, may affect many joints. Pain may be progressive, as in ankylosing spondylitis, or the patient may experience simultaneous inflammation in multiple joints, as in rheumatic fever. Arthralgia joint pain unaccompanied by heat, redness, and swelling is a common vague complaint in many infections.

Joint pain commonly occurs in rheumatoid arthritis, systemic lupus erythematosus, progressive systemic sclerosis, inflammatory bowel disease, and acute rheumatic fever. Other autoimmune rheumatic disorders that cause joint pain include polymyositis with dermatomyositis, ankylosing spondylitis, Reiter's syndrome, Behçet's syndrome, and mixed connective tissue disease.

If your patient complains of joint pain, take his health history and perform a physical examination according to the guidelines that follow.

History of the symptom
To further explore your patient's joint pain, consider asking him the following questions:
• When did you first feel joint pain?
• Did the pain occur suddenly? Or did it develop over weeks or months?
• Does the pain involve one joint or several? (Have the patient locate the affected joints.)
• If several, has the pain spread to other joints while remaining in the initial one? Or has it disappeared from the original site?
• How would you describe the type of pain? How would you rate its intensity on a scale of 1 (least severe) to 10 (most severe)?
• At what time of day is your pain worst?
• What makes the pain worse? What helps to relieve it?
• How does the pain affect your ability to carry out daily activities?
• Does it affect your sleep?
• Does it affect your emotional well-being?

Associated findings
Note whether the patient has experienced any of the following signs and symptoms:
• joint stiffness or deformity
• joint warmth, redness, and swelling
• limitation of movement
• fever with or without chills
• fatigue
• anorexia
• weight loss
• muscle weakness
• lymphadenopathy
• skin lesions
• sore throat
• diarrhea
• abdominal pain
• urinary burning, frequency, or urgency.

Previous conditions and treatments
Consult with the patient, family members, or members of the health care team to determine if the patient has ever had any of the following disorders, risk factors, or treatments:
• trauma
• excessive use of joints
• infection, especially gonorrhea or Lyme disease
• rheumatic disease

• arthroscopy
• joint surgery, including joint replacement.

Drug history
Note past or current use of any of the drugs listed below.
   The following drugs may cause drug-induced arthralgia:
• isotretinoin
• interferon alfa-n3 (derived from human leukocytes)
• lymphocyte immune globulin, antithymocyte globulin (equine)
• epoetin alfa
• nicotine transdermal systems
• etretinate
• naltrexone.
   The following drugs may cause drug-induced lupus-like syndrome with arthralgia:
• hydralazine
• procainamide
• methyldopa
• isoniazid
• cephalosporins
• phenytoin
• quinidine
• sulfonamides
• bleomycin
• oral contraceptives.

Physical examination
Examine the patient according to the steps described below.
• Check the patient's height, weight, and vital signs, including temperature, blood pressure, respiratory rate and depth, and pulse rate and rhythm.
• Note the patient's general appearance and mobility.
• Inspect for signs of joint inflammation, including swelling around the joint and redness of the overlying skin.
• Note the presence of joint deformities, and check for symmetrical involvement. Observe the surrounding area for abnormalities, such as subcutaneous nodules and muscle atrophy.
• Firmly palpate each joint, noting any thickening, swelling, laxity, tenderness, or crepitus.
• Note any limitation in the normal range of joint motion.

• Test the strength of surrounding muscles, noting any weakness.

Let the patient's history and the musculoskeletal assessment findings guide the remainder of the physical examination.

Rash

Rashes and skin lesions are classified as follows:

• Macular lesions, such as petechiae, are less than 1 cm in diameter and are circumscribed and flat.
• A patch is similar to a macular lesion but is larger.
• Papules are palpably elevated solid lesions up to 0.5 cm in diameter.
• Plaque is similar to papules but larger.
• Wheals are irregular, transient, superficial areas of localized skin edema, such as hives.
• Vesicles, which occur in herpes simplex, are circumscribed, superficial, fluid-filled elevations up to 0.5 cm in diameter.
• Bullae, which occur in bullous pemphigoid, are circumscribed superficial elevations greater than 0.5 cm in diameter and filled with serous fluid.
• Pustules, which occur in acne, are circumscribed superficial elevations filled with pus.

Outbreak of a rash may be accompanied by pruritus and discomfort. A rash may profoundly affect the patient's body image.

Rash commonly occurs in acquired immunodeficiency syndrome, infection caused by *Mycobacterium haemophilum,* histoplasmosis, cutaneous T-cell lymphoma, molluscum contagiosum, systemic lupus erythematosus, polymyositis with dermatomyositis, acute rheumatic fever, progressive systemic sclerosis, pemphigus vulgaris, and bullous pemphigoid. Rash also occurs in hypersensitivity reactions, such as serum sickness, allergic reaction to insect bites, anaphylaxis, allergic dermatitis, contact dermatitis, and atopic dermatitis.

If your patient complains of a rash, take his health history and perform a physical examination according to the guidelines that follow.

History of the sign
To further explore the patient's complaint of a rash, consider asking the following questions:
• When did the rash erupt? What did it look like? What parts of your body did it affect?
• Has the rash spread or changed in any way? If so, when and how did it spread?
• Does the rash itch or burn? Is it painful or tender?
• Have you recently been bitten by an insect or a rodent?
• Have you had direct skin contact with known allergens, such as detergents or foods?
• Have you recently been exposed to anyone with an infectious disease?
• Which medications have you recently taken?
• Have you applied any topical agents to the rash and, if so, when was the last application? Were any of them effective?
• What childhood diseases have you had?
• What immunizations have you had?
• How do you feel about the appearance of the rash?

Associated findings
Note if the patient has experienced any of the following signs or symptoms:
• headache
• fever
• cough
• fatigue
• joint pain
• lymphadenopathy
• diarrhea
• urinary burning or frequency
• difficulty breathing, stridor, or wheezing
• unusual bleeding or bruising.

Previous conditions and treatments
Consult with the patient, family members, or members of the health care team to determine if the patient has ever had any of the following disorders, treatments, or risk factors:
• allergies
• recent diagnostic studies using contrast agents
• immunosuppressive therapy
• other skin disorders

• sexually transmitted disease or other infection
• connective tissue disease
• cancer
• trauma.

Drug history
Obtain a drug history. Many drugs can cause rashes; some of the most common include:
• penicillins
• sulfonamides
• aspirin
• barbiturates
• gold compounds
• glucocorticoids
• oral contraceptives
• thiazides
• tetracyclines
• phenylbutazone
• captopril
• enalaprilat
• enalapril maleate
• isocarboxazid
• bleomycin
• lymphocyte immune globulin, antithymocyte globulin (equine)
• allopurinol
• methyldopa
• phenytoin.

Physical examination
Check the patient's height, weight, and vital signs, including temperature, blood pressure, respiratory rate and depth, and pulse rate and rhythm. Then examine the patient according to the steps described below.

Inspection
• Observe the patient's general appearance. Note if he appears in distress and if he's scratching the lesion. Does he appear cachectic, lethargic, listless, or restless and anxious?
• Inspect the patient's skin, noting whether it's dry or oily. Note the anatomic location, general distribution and arrangement, color, shape, and size of the lesions.
• Check for crusts, macules, papules, vesicles, scales, scars, and wheals. Note if the outer layer of epidermis separates easily from the basal layer.

Palpation
• Feel the temperature of the patient's skin, using the back of your fingers. Compare affected and unaffected areas, noting whether they feel cool or hot.
• Palpate vesicles or bullae to determine whether they're flaccid or tense.

Let the patient's history and the dermatologic assessment findings guide the rest of the physical examination.

Common Treatments for Immune Disorders

Bone marrow transplantation

The infusion of fresh or stored bone marrow from a donor to a recipient is known as bone marrow transplantation (BMT). This treatment replaces diseased bone marrow with healthy bone marrow and possibly enables the recipient's body to resume normal production of blood cells. Whether a patient undergoes this transplantation procedure depends on his age and health status, the underlying disease, and the availability of a histocompatible donor.

Types of BMT include autologous (procured from the patient and frozen), syngeneic (procured from the patient's identical twin), and allogeneic (procured from a histocompatible donor). Autologous bone marrow must be thawed immediately before infusion. Syngeneic and allogeneic bone marrow are infused immediately after procurement from the donor.

Although autologous BMT poses the least risk of infection for the recipient, it isn't always a viable option for the patient with diseased bone marrow. Because it doesn't pose a risk of graft-versus-host disease (GVHD), syngeneic BMT poses a lower risk of infection than allogeneic BMT.

Indications
To treat severe combined immunodeficiency disease and acute or chronic leukemia

Complications
• Acute or chronic GVHD (allogeneic BMT)
• Bleeding
• Life-threatening bacterial, viral, and fungal infections
• Hepatic venoocclusive disease, leading to multisystem organ failure

Plasmapheresis

Also known as therapeutic plasma exchange, plasmapheresis involves the removal of plasma from withdrawn blood and the reinfusion of formed blood elements. Treatment may remove up to 90% of unwanted plasma factors, including autoantibodies, immune complexes, metabolites, toxic substances, and unknown mediators of disease.

Indications
To treat autoimmune thrombocytopenic purpura or myasthenia gravis

Complications
• Infection around the venipuncture site
• Hypersensitivity reaction to the ingredients of the replacement solution
• Hypocalcemia from excessive binding of circulating calcium to the citrate solution used as an anticoagulant in the replacement solution
• Arrhythmias
• Hypotension and other complications of low blood volume, such as syncope
• Hypomagnesemia leading to severe muscle cramps, tetany, and paresthesia (may follow repeated plasmapheresis)
• Symptoms of myasthenic crisis, such as dysphagia, ptosis, and diplopia, in patients with myasthenia gravis (secondary to removal of antibodies or antimyasthenic drugs from the blood)
• Hemolysis or embolism (rare)

Radiation therapy

Radiation therapy provides high levels of gamma rays or X-rays through a beam of electrons to a targeted area of cells or tissues.

Indications
To treat severe rheumatoid arthritis or lupus nephritis and to prevent kidney transplant rejection (these indications still under investigation)

Complications
- Interstitial pneumonitis
- Pulmonary fibrosis
- Pulmonary toxicity
- Chronic gastritis or enteritis
- GI bleeding
- Diarrhea
- Intractable nausea
- Vomiting
- Intestinal obstruction
- Oral complications such as stomatitis

- Myelosuppression
- Pericarditis and pericardial effusions
- Cerebral edema with an increased risk of seizures, inflammation, and increased intracranial pressure

Splenectomy

Removal of the spleen (splenectomy) curtails the spleen's role in intercepting antigens or antigenic chemical products that have succeeded in reaching the circulating blood.

Indication
To treat symptomatic hypersplenism associated with such disorders as autoimmune thrombocytopenic purpura or autoimmune hemolytic anemia

Complications
Increased susceptibility to infection, especially with encapsulated bacteria such as *Streptococcus pneumoniae;* high incidence of fulminant, rapidly fatal bacteremia

Common Drugs for Immune Disorders

Immune disorders are commonly treated with anti-inflammatory drugs, immunosuppressants, biological response modifiers, and colony-stimulating factors.

Anti-inflammatory drugs

Corticosteroids
• Short-acting: hydrocortisone, cortisone
• Intermediate-acting: prednisone, prednisolone, triamcinolone, methylprednisolone
• Long-acting: dexamethasone, betamethasone
• Mineralocorticoids: fludrocortisone

Indications
Adrenal insufficiency; systemic or inhalation therapy for respiratory diseases (asthma); relief of inflammation in rheumatoid arthritis and collagen disorders (lupus erythematosus, scleroderma); suppression of inflammatory reactions in asthma, ulcerative colitis, and Crohn's disease; food and drug allergies; emergency treatment of shock and anaphylactic reactions; prevention of rejection in organ and tissue transplants; adjunctive treatment of leukemias, lymphomas, and myelomas; multiple sclerosis; topical treatment of dermatologic and ocular inflammations

Adverse reactions
• CNS: *euphoria, insomnia,* psychotic behavior, pseudotumor cerebri
• CV: edema, hypertension, ***congestive heart failure***
• Endocrine: menstrual irregularities, growth suppression in children, cushingoid signs (moon face, buffalo hump, truncal obesity)
• GI: nausea, vomiting, *peptic ulcer,* ***pancreatitis***
• Metabolic: hyperglycemia, hypocalcemia, hypokalemia
• Other: muscle weakness or myopathy and weakening of the skeletal system due to loss of calcium from bones; acne, hirsutism, impaired wound healing, emotional instability, ophthalmic changes.

Note: Abrupt withdrawal of corticosteroids after long-term use can precipitate potentially fatal adrenal crisis.

Gold salts
Auranofin, aurothioglucose, gold sodium thiomalate

Indications
Progressive rheumatoid arthritis

Adverse reactions
• Blood: ***agranulocytosis, aplastic anemia, thrombocytopenia***
• GI: stomatitis, metallic taste, *nausea, vomiting, abdominal cramps* (especially with auranofin)
• GU: nephrotic syndrome, proteinuria, renal impairment
• Hepatic: hepatitis
• Respiratory: pneumonitis, pulmonary fibrosis
• Skin: *rash, pruritus, dermatitis,* ***exfoliative dermatitis***

NSAIDs
Diclofenac, etodolac, fenoprofen, flurbiprofen, ibuprofen, indomethacin, ketoprofen, ketorolac, meclofenamate, nabumetone, naproxen, piroxicam, sulindac, tolmetin

Indications
Mild to moderate pain, such as myalgia or arthralgia; inflammation due to rheumatoid arthritis or other inflammatory disorders (used with an opioid analgesic for severe pain); short-term postoperative analgesia (I.M. ketorolac)

Common reactions are in *italics;* life-threatening reactions in ***bold italics.***

Adverse reactions
- Blood: *prolonged bleeding time*
- GI: *GI upset, heartburn, nausea, vomiting,* **peptic ulcer,** bleeding
- GU: acute renal failure
- Hepatic: **hepatotoxicity**
- Other: **bronchospasm, anaphylaxis** (in aspirin-allergic patients)

Nonopioid analgesics
Acetaminophen, salicylates (aspirin, choline magnesium trisalicylate, choline salicylate, diflunisal, salsalate, sodium salicylate)

Indications for acetaminophen
Mild to moderate pain; preferable to aspirin or NSAIDs for pain if patient has a history of GI bleeding, peptic ulcer, or aspirin or NSAID intolerance

Adverse reactions to acetaminophen
- Hepatic: **hepatic necrosis** (with high doses)
- Skin: rash, urticaria
- Other: angioedema, **anaphylaxis** (rare)

Indications for salicylates
Mild to moderate pain, such as myalgia or arthralgia; inflammation due to rheumatoid arthritis or other inflammatory disorders (used with an opioid analgesic for severe pain)

Adverse reactions to salicylates
- Blood: *prolonged bleeding time,* **blood dyscrasias**
- CNS: headache, dizziness, confusion, lassitude, drowsiness (in patients taking diflunisal)
- CV: tachycardia
- EENT: *tinnitus, hearing loss,* dim vision
- GI: *dyspepsia, heartburn, epigastric distress, nausea, abdominal pain*
- Hepatic: **hepatotoxicity**
- Respiratory: **bronchospasm** (with or without angiospasm), hyperventilation
- Other: sweating, renal damage, **hypersensitivity manifested as anaphylaxis or, with aspirin, as asthma**

Immunosuppressants

Azathioprine

Indications
Inflammatory diseases, such as rheumatoid arthritis, psoriatic arthritis, and systemic lupus erythematosus; prevention of organ rejection after transplant surgery

Adverse reactions
- Blood: anemia, **bone marrow suppression, thrombocytopenia,** leukopenia
- CV: pulmonary fibrosis
- GI: nausea, vomiting, anorexia, **pancreatitis**
- Hepatic: elevated liver enzyme levels
- Other: **immunosuppression,** arthralgia, muscle weakness

Cyclophosphamide

Indications
Inflammatory diseases, such as rheumatoid arthritis, psoriatic arthritis, and systemic lupus erythematosus; cancer

Adverse reactions
- Blood: anemia, **bone marrow suppression, thrombocytopenia,** leukopenia
- CV: pulmonary fibrosis
- GI: nausea, vomiting, **pancreatitis**
- Hepatic: elevated liver enzyme levels

Cyclosporine

Indications
Prevention of organ rejection after transplant surgery; also used with corticosteroids to reduce inflammation in rheumatoid arthritis

Adverse reactions
- CNS: *tremor,* headache
- GI: *gum hyperplasia,* nausea, vomiting, diarrhea, abdominal distention
- GU: **nephrotoxicity**
- Hepatic: **hepatotoxicity**

Common reactions are in *italics;* life-threatening reactions in **bold italics.**

• Metabolic: hyperkalemia, hyperglycemia
• Other: hypertension, *hirsutism,* sinusitis, gynecomastia, hearing loss, tinnitus, muscle pain, edema

Hydroxychloroquine

Indications
Severe rheumatoid arthritis and systemic lupus erythematosus; suppression and chemoprophylaxis of malaria

Adverse reactions
• Blood: *aplastic anemia, thrombocytopenia,* leukopenia
• CNS: irritability, headache, dizziness
• GI: anorexia, nausea, vomiting, cramps
• Skin: bleaching of hair, alopecia, skin eruptions, pruritus
• Other: *hypersensitivity* (dermatitis, urticaria, angioedema), retinopathy

Lymphocyte immune globulin

Indications
Rescue therapy in transplant rejection; mild or severe aplastic anemia

Adverse reactions
• Blood: leukopenia, thrombocytopenia
• CNS: malaise, seizures, headache
• Other: fever, chills, skin reactions

Methotrexate

Indications
Inflammatory diseases, such as rheumatoid arthritis, psoriatic arthritis, vasculitis, inflammatory bowel disease, and systemic lupus erythematosus; cancer

Adverse reactions
• Blood: anemia, *bone marrow suppression, thrombocytopenia,* leukopenia
• CV: pulmonary fibrosis
• GI: nausea, vomiting, *pancreatitis*
• Hepatic: elevated liver enzyme levels

Muromonab-CD3

Indications
Reversal of acute renal allograft rejection (not effective as a single-agent prophylaxis)

Adverse reactions
• Blood: pancytopenia, *aplastic anemia,* neutropenia
• CV: *cardiac arrest,* hypotension, shock
• GI: *nausea, vomiting,* diarrhea
• GU: renal dysfunction
• Respiratory: *respiratory arrest, acute respiratory distress syndrome, pulmonary edema*
• Skin: rash, urticaria, flushing, pruritus
• Other: *fever, chills,* dyspnea, headache

Penicillamine

Indications
Inflammatory diseases, such as rheumatoid arthritis, psoriatic arthritis, and systemic lupus erythematosus

Adverse reactions
• Blood: *bone marrow suppression, thrombocytopenia,* leukopenia
• EENT: tinnitus, *reversible optic neuritis*
• GI: anorexia, epigastric pain, nausea, vomiting, stomatitis, loss of taste
• GU: proteinuria, *nephrotic syndrome*
• Other: *allergic reactions* (pruritus, rash), lupus-like syndrome

Tacrolimus

Indications
Rescue therapy in liver transplant recipients with failing grafts who are receiving cyclosporine-based immunosuppressive therapy (investigational)

Adverse reactions
(Most prevalent with I.V. tacrolimus and during combined use with cyclosporine)

Common reactions are in *italics;* life-threatening reactions in **bold italics.**

- CNS: neurotoxicity (headache, tremor, paresthesia, photophobia, tinnitus, sleep disturbances, mood changes)
- Other: *nephrotoxicity,* hypertension, GI disturbances, impaired glucose tolerance

Biological response modifiers and colony-stimulating factors

Aldesleukin

Indications
Metastatic renal cell cancer

Adverse reactions
- Blood: *anemia, **thrombocytopenia,*** leukopenia, coagulation disorders, leukocytosis, eosinophilia
- CNS: *mental status changes* (lethargy, somnolence, confusion, agitation), *dizziness, syncope, motor dysfunction, **coma***
- CV: capillary leak syndrome leading to hypotension, occasional arrhythmias
- GI: *nausea, vomiting, diarrhea, stomatitis, anorexia, bleeding, dyspepsia, constipation*
- GU: **oliguria, anuria,** *proteinuria, hematuria, dysuria,* urine retention, urinary frequency
- Hepatic: *elevated liver enzyme levels, jaundice, hepatomegaly*
- Respiratory: **pulmonary edema, respiratory failure**
- Skin: *pruritus, erythema, rash,* **exfoliative dermatitis**
- Other: **sepsis**

Epoetin alfa

Indications
Anemia secondary to reduced production of endogenous erythropoietin; anemia secondary to end-stage renal disease; adjunctive treatment of patients infected with human immunodeficiency virus and anemia secondary to zidovudine (or other antiretroviral) therapy

Adverse reactions
- Blood: iron deficiency, elevated platelet count
- CNS: headache, **seizures**
- CV: *hypertension,* clotting of the vascular access device and increased clotting in arteriovenous grafts, tachycardia
- GI: nausea, vomiting, diarrhea
- Metabolic: hyperkalemia
- Skin: rash

Filgrastim

Indications
Reduction in duration and severity of chemotherapy-induced myelosuppression and increased circulating neutrophil counts; may allow administration of higher doses of chemotherapeutic drugs

Adverse reactions
- Blood: **thrombocytopenia**
- GU: hematuria, proteinuria
- Skin: alopecia, exacerbation of preexisting skin conditions (such as psoriasis)
- Other: bone pain and erythema at injection site; reversible elevations in levels of uric acid, lactate dehydrogenase, and alkaline phosphatase; *skeletal pain,* fever, splenomegaly, osteoporosis

Interferon alfa-2a, recombinant; interferon alfa-2b, recombinant

Indications
- Interferon alfa-2a: hairy-cell leukemia, Kaposi's sarcoma related to acquired immunodeficiency syndrome (AIDS)
- Interferon alfa-2b: hairy-cell leukemia; Kaposi's sarcoma related to AIDS; chronic hepatitis; condylomata acuminata

Adverse reactions
- Blood: **leukopenia,** mild thrombocytopenia
- CNS: *dizziness,* confusion, paresthesia, lethargy, depression, nervousness, irritability, *fatigue*
- CV: hypotension or hypertension, chest pain, arrhythmias, **congestive heart failure** (alfa-2a), edema, neutropenia

Common reactions are in *italics;* life-threatening reactions in **bold italics.**

- GI: anorexia, nausea, vomiting, *diarrhea*
- Respiratory: *bronchospasm* (alfa-2a), coughing, dyspnea
- Skin: *rash,* dry skin, *pruritus,* partial alopecia, urticaria
- Other: pharyngitis, *flulike symptoms* (fever, headache, chills, muscle aches), elevated liver enzyme levels

Interferon alfa-n3

Indications
Condylomata acuminata

Adverse reactions
- Blood: neutropenia
- CNS: dizziness, light-headedness
- GI: anorexia, dyspepsia, nausea, vomiting
- Hepatic: elevated liver enzyme levels
- Skin: rash, pruritus, partial alopecia
- Other: *constitutional or flulike symptoms* (fever, myalgia, headache, chills, malaise, arthralgia)

Interferon gamma-1b

Indications
Reduction of frequency and severity of infections associated with chronic granulomatous disease

Adverse reactions
- CV: occasional (dose-related) hypotension
- GI: diarrhea, nausea, vomiting
- Skin: rash

Interleukin-3, recombinant human

Indications
Early stem cell precursor to G-CSF or GM-CSF with possible role in treating leukemia, refractory anemia, and myelodysplastic syndromes, and combined with GM-CSF following autologous bone marrow transplant (investigational)

Adverse reactions
Mild constitutional symptoms

Macrophage colony-stimulating factor

Indications
Potent inducer of monocytosis; may enhance direct cytotoxicity against tumor targets for some cancers (investigational)

Adverse reactions
- Blood: mild thrombocytopenia, decreased low-density lipoprotein levels

Sargramostim

Indications
Reduction in duration and severity of chemotherapy-induced myelosuppression and increased circulating neutrophil counts in patients with myelodysplastic syndromes, aplastic anemia, or agranulocytosis and in recipients of bone marrow transplants

Adverse reactions
- Blood: *blood dyscrasia*
- CNS: fatigue, malaise, CNS disorder
- CV: hemorrhage
- GI: nausea, vomiting, diarrhea, anorexia, hemorrhage, stomatitis, liver damage
- GU: urinary tract disorders, renal dysfunction
- Respiratory: dyspnea, lung disorders
- Skin: alopecia, rash
- Local: erythema at injection site
- Other: bone pain, edema, fever, *sepsis*

Tumor necrosis factor

Indications
AIDS, cancers (investigational), sepsis (investigational)

Adverse reactions
- Blood: anemia, neutropenia, hypertriglyceridemia
- CNS: fatigue, malaise
- CV: hypotension
- GI: anorexia
- Hepatic: elevated liver enzyme levels
- Metabolic: hyperglycemia
- Other: fever, flulike symptoms

Common reactions are in *italics*; life-threatening reactions in ***bold italics.***

ICD-9-CM Classification of Immune Disorders

The *International Classification of Diseases,* 9th revision, *Clinical Modification (ICD-9-CM),* standardizes the classification of immune disorders. In this classification, you'll find these abbreviations:

NOS = not otherwise specified
NEC = not elsewhere classifed.

---

279 Immune disorders

279.0 Deficiency of humoral immunity
  279.00 Hypogammaglobulinemia, unspecified
  Agammaglobulinemia NOS
  279.01 Selective immunoglobulin A (IgA) immunodeficiency
  279.02 Selective immunoglobulin (IgM) immunodeficiency
  279.03 Other selective immunoglobulin deficiencies:
  Selective deficiency of immunoglobulin G (IgG)
  279.04 Congenital hypogammaglobulinemia
  Agammaglobulinemia:
    Bruton's type
    X-linked
  279.05 Immunodeficiency with increased IgM
  Immunodeficiency with hyper-IgM:
    autosomal recessive
    X-linked
  279.06 Common variable immunodeficiency
  Dysgammaglobulinemia (acquired, congenital, or primary)
  Hypogammaglobulinemia:
    acquired
    primary
    congenital, not sex-linked
    sporadic

279.09 Other
  Transient hypogammaglobulinemia of infancy

279.1 Deficiency of cell-mediated immunity
  279.10 Immunodeficiency with predominant T-cell defect, unspecified
  279.11 DiGeorge's syndrome
  Pharyngeal pouch syndrome
  Thymic hypoplasia
  279.12 Wiskott-Aldrich syndrome
  279.13 Nezelof syndrome
  Cellular immunodeficiency with abnormal immunoglobulin deficiency
  279.19 Other
  Excludes ataxia-telangiectasia (334.8)

279.2 Combined immunity deficiency
  Agammaglobulinemia:
    autosomal recessive
    Swiss-type
    X-linked recessive
  Severe combined immunodeficiency
  Thymic:
    alymphoplasia
    aplasia or dysplasia with immunodeficiency
  Excludes thymic hypoplasia (279.11)

279.3 Unspecified immunity deficiency

279.4 Autoimmune disease NEC
  Autoimmune disease NOS
  Excludes transplant failure or rejection (996.80 to 996.89)

279.8 Other immune disorders
  Single complement (C1 to C9) deficiency or dysfunction

279.9 Unspecified immune disorder

Index

i refers to an illustration; t refers to a table

i refers to an illustration; t refers to a table

i refers to an illustration; t refers to a table

i refers to an illustration; t refers to a table

i refers to an illustration; t refers to a table

i refers to an illustration; t refers to a table

i refers to an illustration; t refers to a table

i refers to an illustration; t refers to a table

i refers to an illustration; t refers to a table